Transcultural Nursing
Theory and Models

Priscilla Limbo Sagar, EdD, RN, ACNS-BC, CTN-A, is a professor of nursing at Mount Saint Mary College in Newburgh, New York. She received a BS in Nursing from the Philippine Women's University; an MS in Adult Nursing, minor in education from Pace University; and an EdD in nursing education/professorial role from Teachers College, Columbia University. She is board certified in adult health from the American Nurses Credentialing Center and has advanced certification from the Transcultural Nursing Society. Her research interests include international nursing, mentoring, partnerships and collaborations, and transcultural nursing (TCN). She serves as consultant in the areas of cultural diversity and promotion of cultural competence as well as in curriculum development, implementation, and evaluation. In addition, Dr. Sagar had facilitated several national and international conferences to disseminate TCN research and knowledge. She is a longtime member of the Transcultural Nursing Society and chairs the Eligibility and Credentialing Committee of the Transcultural Nursing Certification Commission. Dr. Sagar also teaches as an adjunct faculty for University of Phoenix Online's School of Advanced Studies where she has assisted in dissertations with cultural diversity and transcultural focus.

TRANSCULTURAL NURSING THEORY AND MODELS

Application in Nursing Education, Practice, and Administration

Priscilla Limbo Sagar, EdD, RN, ACNS-BC, CTN-A

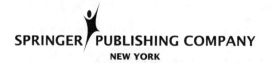

SPRINGER PUBLISHING COMPANY

NEW YORK

Springer Publishing Company, LLC
11 West 42nd Street
New York, NY 10036
www.springerpub.com

Acquisitions Editor: Allan Graubard
Production Editor: Dana Bigelow
Composition: Newgen Imaging

ISBN: 978–0–8261–0748–0
E-book ISBN: 978–0–8261–0749–7

11 12 13/5 4 3 2 1

The author and the publisher of this Work have made every effort to use sources believed to be reliable to provide information that is accurate and compatible with the standards generally accepted at the time of publication. The author and publisher shall not be liable for any special, consequential, or exemplary damages resulting, in whole or in part, from the readers' use of, or reliance on, the information contained in this book. The publisher has no responsibility for the persistence or accuracy of URLs for external or third-party Internet Web sites referred to in this publication and does not guarantee that any content on such Web sites is, or will remain, accurate or appropriate.

Library of Congress Cataloging-in-Publication Data
Sagar, Priscilla Limbo.
  Transcultural nursing theory and models : application in nursing education, practice, and administration / Priscilla Limbo Sagar.
    p. ; cm.
Includes bibliographical references and index.
ISBN 978-0-8261-0748-0 — ISBN 978-0-8261-0749-7 (e-book)
1. Transcultural nursing. 2. Nursing models. I. Title.
[DNLM: 1. Transcultural Nursing. 2. Models, Nursing.
3. Nursing Theory. WY 107]
RT86.54.S24 2012
610.73—dc23   2011026505

Printed in the United States of America by Gasch Printing.

This book is dedicated to

My loving family: husband Drew Sagar for his unconditional love and support; daughter Alexa, and grandson Andrew Michael; parents Trinidad and Mercedes Limbo and family; and to my late mother-in-law Joy Sagar-Radomski.

Dr. Madeline Leininger, founder and leader of transcultural nursing, for her tireless, courageous, and untiring effort for six decades in building transcultural nursing knowledge and for her laborious work on behalf of TCN.

Other pioneering transcultural nurses who contributed, are contributing, and will contribute to the field of TCN. Because of Dr. Leininger and these nurses, we have a wealth of knowledge for evidence-based practice in transcultural nursing. Past mentors at Teachers College, Columbia University: Dr. Sheila O. Melli, Dr. Marie O'Toole, and Dr. Caroline Camuñas.

CONTENTS

FOREWORD

Madeleine M. Leininger, PhD, LHD, DS, RN, CTN, FAAN, LL
Founder of Transcultural Nursing
and
Leader in Culture Care Theory and Research

One of the most significant and revolutionary movements in nursing and the health fields during the past six decades has been the theoretical, intellectual, and research studies for educators and professional leaders to understand culture and then incorporate cultural content into health services. This new body of transcultural nursing and caring knowledge is held to initiate and to improve the quality of care to people of diverse and similar cultures. This has been a major and significant movement led by myself and a few committed nurses to incorporate holistic, broad, specific, and general culture care concepts into health services. The incorporation of culture care principles and theoretical research findings into health care practices by teaching and applying transculturally based health care has been emphasized. The movement began in the late 1970s when I realized the cultural dimensions bearing upon understanding and helping people of diverse cultures were major and missing dimensions in health care. It was through repeated direct observations that I discovered the absence of cultural factors in people care. There were missing factors influencing illness, health, wellness, recovery, and health maintenance. I chose to be a leader to change this long neglected area in nursing and health care. I also chose to stimulate other health disciplines to work toward this goal.

Initially, this ambitious leadership goal seemed overwhelming and impossible with limited resources and virtually no prepared faculty to teach and conduct research related to bringing culture into health care practices. However, the need for change was great and the benefits to clients seemed most promising and important. Hence, the challenges and benefits were noteworthy.

From the beginning, I held that the nursing profession with its central focus on human care could play a central role to make transcultural care possible and a substantive focus of a new field I called transcultural nursing and health care. Persistence, diligence, and creative leadership were needed to achieve this major goal and bring changes into health care. I began this movement by emphasizing the educational preparation of undergraduate and graduate nurse students into the new field of transcultural nursing study and practice. Almost immediately, I discovered that nursing students became highly motivated and excited about the actual and potential benefits of nurses to establish this new role and practice in nursing. The course content was stimulating to them and the idea spread to many nurses and health care providers who became interested to learn about culturally based care. Then I discovered that the master and doctoral nursing students were interested in transcultural nursing and wanted to be prepared in the new field. These undergraduate and graduate students led the way to make transcultural nursing a reality. They became active supporters to promote transcultural nursing care with and for cultures. These were most encouraging factors and helped carve the pathway to establish the new field of transcultural nursing. The students' enthusiasm and vision of transcultural health care as a new field of study and practice in nursing were noteworthy.

In the mid-1960s I realized my need for doctoral preparation in anthropology and pursued doctoral study in cultural and social anthropology. Then I encouraged other nurses to follow similar preparation in order to assure in-depth knowledge of cultures. These practices opened the door for nurses, physicians, and other health professionals to study Western and non-Western cultures with a comparative focus. I was particularly interested to discover culturally based care meanings, expressions, and care practices of cultures to realize the vast wealth of untapped cultural knowledge available to study and apply to health care with a comparative focus.

By the early 1960s, human care with a transcultural focus became known and the pathway for transcultural health research became apparent to nurses and other health care practitioners, providers, and researchers. Soon the traditional focus in nursing on medical diseases, symptoms, and treatment modes was decreased and transcultural care became the central interest. Culturally based care with cultural care meanings, uses, practices to heal, and to maintain well-being began to be emphasized by the late 1970s.

It was the development of my Theory of Culture Care Diversity and Universality that stimulated and guided many students and others to discover culture care *diversities* and *universalities*. The theory was an important guide to help investigators to enter the world of culture and to learn directly from the people about their culture. I developed and encouraged the use of qualitative research methods to tease out culture care data with the use of the ethnonursing method. This method had five ways to help investigators identify care meanings and their uses in specific cultures. It was the development and use of the *Sunrise Enabler* as a conceptual guide for students and researchers to grasp the scope and areas to obtain transcultural nursing data. Using the Sunrise model, students could identify appropriate decisions and actions for the application of therapeutic culturally based care. Thus, both the theory and method were essential to discover and apply transcultural nursing knowledge.

This brief overview to discover transcultural nursing took nearly 50 years to obtain and understand Western and non-Western cultural knowledge. This was an exciting and noteworthy time as students teased out the subtle, covert cultural phenomena as the new transcultural nursing care knowledge. Since then and today, transcultural nursing has become established with many nurse researchers and health professionals using this knowledge to care for cultures. Today, health care providers can provide care that is congruent or appropriate to specific cultures in accord with their cultural values and lifeways. Transcultural care has become a reality and is welcomed by many clients with positive benefits in health care, recovery, and well being. Many clients have told the author and others that providing transcultural nursing care is greatly valued and essential to them. For example, several older clients told the author, "I never thought this kind of care would occur in my lifetime. It is a joy and so helpful to me and my culture because it fits my lifeways. Thank you."

I believe this book by Priscilla Limbo Sagar offers a further step to advance, strengthen, support, and sustain the new transcultural nursing field and health care in general. The author offers models and visual aids to assess, apply, and use transcultural nursing and related findings for improved care. Such aids in learning and practice can be used in addition to current knowledge and existing methods. These models can be helpful to build transcultural and other nursing care knowledge to transform health care practices.

I believe this book with a major focus on assessment and use of transcultural nursing theory and research findings will lead to a wealth of new principles, practices, and policies to guide health care providers for quality care services to cultures. This knowledge should build upon existing knowledge and provide choices and guides to practice. Such contributions will not only build and strengthen health care and transcultural nursing but should help guide practitioners to become global and skillful practitioners as we expand and serve people of many cultures in the world.

I believe this book will be helpful to nurses, especially baccalaureate and graduate students, as well as to interdisciplinary health students and practitioners to envision and discover many creative and effective approaches to know, understand, and serve cultures. Having new and explicated content, models, and guides will enable practitioners to move forward transcultural health care into new discoveries and beneficial ways to health and wellness. It will also help to avoid cultural biases, prejudices, destructive practices, and cultural ignorance. Moreover, transcultural nursing practice will become essential to provide quality-based health services in the near future. In the early 1960s, it was my hope that by this 21st century, health values, beliefs, and practices of most cultures would be known and fully understood, and practitioners would be able to skillfully and knowingly apply knowledge that is tailored to cultures to maintain their health care and well-being. Thus, by using appropriate theories, models, research methods, and research findings, a wealth of creative new knowledge and practices will be forthcoming.

Today, there are several transcultural nursing books, guides, principles, and research findings with practices that are focused on transcultural nursing to help newcomers and established practitioners provide culturally based nursing and health care. Newcomers can use and build upon existing knowledge and they can expand upon and reaffirm knowledge through practices based on current findings. This will greatly advance practices and assure quality-based health care services. Before long, one can anticipate that transcultural nursing with a holistic and comprehensive comparative focus on culture care will become essential, imperative, and will be required for all health practitioners to be considered professional and safe practitioners. These will be expected norms for licensure of physicians, nurses, and all health care providers. Teachers, practitioners, and administrators will be expected to use transcultural nursing-based knowledge to provide professional services. When this occurs, we will witness major transformations greatly valued by cultures. These developments will be important for the *globalization of transcultural nursing* and quality-based health care as the desired goal of all cultures worldwide.

I believe the author of this book envisioned this goal by stressing the importance of culture care assessments, diverse models, and thera-peutic applications of theory-based research findings that need to be woven into care practices. Before this 21st century ends, global health care will have a significant impact on the quality of health care services rendered not only to cultures in Western and non-Western societies but also to all aspects of humanitarian care. These developments are most promising and possible if health care professionals are *educated* and *prepared* with these goals in mind. The extent of care *diversity* and *universals* as predicted in my Theory of Culture Care Diversity and Universality will become known and will transform health adminis-tration, national and local health policies. Such major contributions to health care will revolutionize and transform health care practices to not only improve and change health services but also become greatly valued and established as desired standards of care. They will become an imperative for cultural, social justice, and humanitarian health care practices for and with cultures. My dream and the dream of futuristic health care providers will be realized.

It is important to state that in the future we will have many books, research projects, and applications of transcultural nursing and of new practices in health care services, practices not realized today. Such con-tributions will help to affirm existing transcultural nursing and new knowledge in health care. They will, indeed, revolutionize current practices in teaching, research, and in administrative policies in many cultures. Cultures can then rejoice that their culture needs will, at last, be recognized and respected, known, understood, and practiced.

Such major revolutions and transformations in health care educa-tion, services, and in administrative practices will be evident world-wide. Such revolutions necessitate change in education, practice, and administration, which this book addresses. It also means we must be committed to culture care with a global vision and commitment. This book by Priscilla L. Sagar should be an important means to reach this goal. In time, the full credibility and realization of transcultural nursing by accurate assessments and the application of research findings from the Culture Care Theory and related theories will yield many benefits. The author is, therefore, to be commended in providing this book to guide nurses and other health care providers toward this goal so that culturally based care with benefits to cultural recipients can be a reality to their health and well-being. Most of all, this book should stimulate readers to think of different ways of using appropriate models, theories, and research methods to guide their thinking and practice. As a consequence, these explorers will find a wealth of new and untapped knowledge to guide their thinking and practice. One can predict they will see the many benefits to health care services between the clients of different and similar cultures.

This book should broaden, expand, and deepen health care in general, and specifically to diverse cultures worldwide. With such refinements of knowledge for culture-specific and cultural universals comparative dimensions of cultures will become evident. The diverse health care needs and practices will be welcome knowledge to health care providers and nurse practitioners, teachers, and researchers to grasp a holistic perspective of ways of knowing, respecting, and understanding cultures. Hopefully, and ultimately, one might anticipate that cultural justice, human care, and health care refinements will be forthcoming and valued as an essential outcome to benefit cultures and the health care providers who have been part of this evolution in health care services. A life with challenges, changes, and beneficial outcomes is always a life worth experiencing and knowing. The time is now to heed those challenges and changes for the transformation of health care. It is what the public is expecting, today and in the future. Most of all, cultures will be respected and valued in teaching, research, practice, administration, and relevant public policies. This will be a great reward for all participants in this endeavor.

REFERENCES

Leininger, M. M., & McFarland, M. R. (2006). *Culture Care Diversity and Universality: A worldwide nursing theory* (2nd ed.). New York, NY: Jones and Bartlett.

Leininger, M. M., & M. McFarland, M. R. (2002). *Transcultural nursing: Concepts, theories, research and practice.* (2nd ed.). New York, NY: McGraw Hill Companies (AJN Book of Year Award 2002).

Leininger, M. M. (1995). *Transcultural nursing: Concepts, theories, research, and practices* (1st ed.). Originally published in 1978, New York: John Wiley & Sons. Reprinted In 1998, Columbus, OH: Greyden Press.

FOREWORD

Margaret M. Andrews, PhD, RN, CTN, FAAN
Director and Professor of Nursing
School of Health Professions and Studies
University of Michigan-Flint;
Editor
Online Journal of Cultural Competence in Nursing and Healthcare

Dr. Priscilla Limbo Sagar's *Transcultural Nursing Theory and Models: Application in Nursing Education, Practice, and Administration* provides a comprehensive, in-depth examination of transcultural healthcare theory and models and critically examines their applications in nursing education, nursing practice, and nursing administration. Dr. Sagar begins this groundbreaking book by presenting Madeleine Leininger's *Theory of Culture Care Diversity and Universality.* The foundress of transcultural nursing, Dr. Leininger created, continuously developed, refined, and evaluated her *Theory of Culture Care Diversity and Universality* during the past six decades using research on hundreds of cultures and subcultures worldwide. Dr. Sagar has crafted a scholarly overview of Leininger's theory, *Sunrise Enabler*, ethnonursing research method, and Leininger's other work in the area of culture care that has influenced the ongoing development of transcultural healthcare and nursing and the creators of the models and guides presented in the remaining chapters of the book.

Dr. Sagar has provided a systematic review of contemporary transcultural healthcare and nursing models such as *Purnell's Model of Cultural Competence*, Campinha-Bacote's *The Process of Cultural Competence in the Delivery of Healthcare Services* and *Biblically Based Model of Cultural Competence*, Giger and Davidhizar's *Transcultural*

Assessment Model, Spector's *Health Traditions Model*, and the Andrews/ Boyle *Nursing Assessment Guide for Individuals and Families*. After reviewing the primary components of the authors' work, Dr. Sagar skillfully crafts conceptual links as she explores applications of theory and models in nursing education, practice, and administration. She also poses NCLEX-type test questions and engages in a constructively critical analysis of the key aspects of the theory and models. Dr. Sagar then invites the reader to a scholarly discussion across the theory and models and called nurses to action as proactive change agents for providing culturally congruent care to people and for promoting culturally competent organizations. She concludes the book with a reflective, thought-provoking look into the future.

Dr. Sagar's work is a must-read synthesis and analysis of the work of key leaders in transcultural healthcare and nursing. She has created a conceptually clear, comprehensive compendium for all health and nursing professionals who are serious about transcultural healthcare models/guides and their applications in nursing education, practice, and administration. Dr. Sagar has made a substantive and important contribution to the advancement of knowledge about transcultural healthcare in this book by clearly explicating and demonstrating the relevance of the theory and models in nursing education, practice, and administration. Dr. Sagar's conceptual linkages to education will assure that the next generation of nurses will graduate from educational programs with curricula rooted in a solid transcultural foundation. Applications to nursing practice will assure that those engaged in the clinical practice of nursing and healthcare will have state-of-the-art knowledge that will enable them to provide culturally congruent and competent care to individuals, groups, and communities from diverse and similar backgrounds. Applications to nursing administration will enable leaders of healthcare organizations, institutions, and agencies to integrate transcultural theory and models into their strategic planning, policies and procedures, responses to national and state accreditation criteria, and related initiatives, thus facilitating organizational cultural competence.

Dr. Sagar is to be congratulated for her outstanding contribution to transcultural healthcare and nursing and to the provision of culturally competent and congruent care for all people.

PREFACE

This book focuses on the application of a transcultural (TCN) nursing theory, four healthcare models, and an assessment guide in nursing education, practice, and administration. Although there is increasing body of knowledge from TCN research spearheaded by Dr. Madeleine Leininger, there is paucity of literature applying those models. More than ever, application in the above fields of nursing is needed to provide (1) nurse educators more resources in integrating cultural competence in nursing curricula; (2) practicing nurses some guidelines to develop culturally congruent care; and (3) nurse leaders various tools to use in innovative approaches for maintaining individual and organizational cultural competence.

Diverse healthcare workers providing care to an increasingly diverse population demand a comprehensive approach to understanding TCN theory and models and their application to education, practice, and administration settings. The discussions under each theory, model, or assessment guide branch out to include current guidelines, mandates, and standards with regard to cultural diversity and promotion of cultural competence. Furthermore, the overlapping between education, practice, and administration is evident—illustrating the dynamic connection between these three realms—in health promotion and in providing equal, safe, and quality healthcare. While there is mention of transcultural research and evidence-based practice, a separate chapter in research application for each theory, model, or assessment guide is beyond the focus of this book.

This book is organized into seven chapters. Six chapters examine one transcultural (TCN) nursing theory, four healthcare models, and an assessment guide: Leininger's *Theory of Culture Care Diversity and Universality*; Purnell's *Model for Cultural Competence*; Campinha-Bacote's *The Process of Cultural Competence in the Delivery of Healthcare Services* and *Biblically Based Model of Cultural Competence in the Delivery of Healthcare Services*; Giger and Davidhizar's *Transcultural Assessment Model*; Spector's *Health Traditions Model*; and Andrews/Boyle *Transcultural Nursing Assessment Guide for Individuals and Families*. Chapter 7 calls nurses—as the largest group of healthcare professionals—to action, and critically examines how their academic, clinical practice, and organizational settings contribute to cultural competence and how each setting could work in harmony and synchrony with mandates and guidelines from the government, accrediting agencies, and professional nursing organizations.

National Council Licensing Examination (NCLEX)–type questions to assist in reviewing and applying key concepts of the theory, models, and assessment guide are placed at the end of Chapters 1 through Chapter 6. These questions will guide nursing educators in integrating cultural diversity and promotion of cultural competence in nursing curricula. In nursing practice, the NCLEX questions will be helpful in applying theory, model, and guide in the assessment, planning, implementation, and evaluation of client care tools and staff development programs.

In addition to the assessment guide, the book uses the five nursing models cited by the American Association of Colleges of Nursing (AACN, 2008) *Cultural Competency in Baccalaureate Nursing Education:* Leininger, Purnell, Campinha-Bacote, Giger and Davidhizar, and Spector. The *Giger and Davidhizar's Model* is used as framework by the National League of Nursing (2009) in the preparation of its *Diversity Toolkit*.

Transcultural Nursing Theory and Models

MADELEINE LEININGER'S THEORY OF CULTURE CARE DIVERSITY AND UNIVERSALITY

SECTION 1. REVIEW OF THE THEORY

Dr. Leininger, the founder and "mother" of transcultural nursing (TCN; Ryan, 2011), started the development of the culture care diversity and universality (CCDU) theory in the late 1940s. According to Glittenberg (2004), Leininger, along with her followers, contributed more than 400 scientific studies to the field of TCN. The founder of TCN pioneered research among the New Guinea Gadsup people; this and her other research became the cornerstone of the CCDU theory (Ryan, 2011). The opening on April 16, 2010, of the Madeleine Leininger Collection on Human Caring and Transcultural Nursing in the Archives of Caring and Nursing at the Christine Lynn College of Nursing, Florida Atlantic University, Boca Raton, Florida, celebrated a life of creativity, courage, and commitment to TCN (Ryan, 2011). Leininger's work in 6 decades established TCN as a formal area of study and discipline in nursing (Andrews, 2008) and instituted its theoretical foundation (Glittenberg, 2004; Ryan, 2011).

Sunrise Enabler to Discover Culture Care

Leininger's theory is depicted as the *sunrise enabler to discover culture care* (Figure 1.1), symbolic of the hope to generate new knowledge for nursing. The model shows factors such as (1) *technological,* (2) *religious and philosophical,* (3) *kinship and social,* (4) *cultural values and lifeways,*

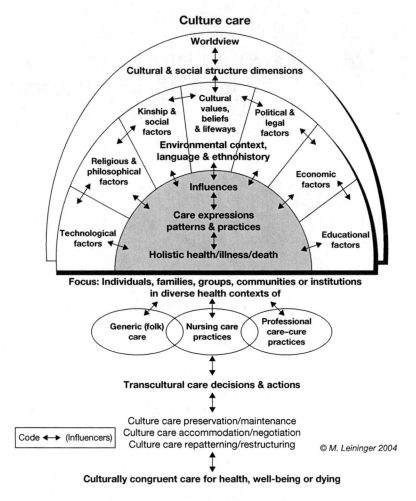

Culture care

Worldview

Cultural & social structure dimensions

Kinship & social factors

Cultural values, beliefs & lifeways

Political & legal factors

Environmental context, language & ethnohistory

Religious & philosophical factors

Economic factors

Influences

Care expressions patterns & practices

Technological factors

Educational factors

Holistic health/illness/death

Focus: Individuals, families, groups, communities or institutions in diverse health contexts of

Generic (folk) care — Nursing care practices — Professional care–cure practices

Transcultural care decisions & actions

Culture care preservation/maintenance
Culture care accommodation/negotiation
Culture care repatterning/restructuring

Code ◄──► (Influencers)

© M. Leininger 2004

Culturally congruent care for health, well-being or dying

FIGURE 1.1 Sunrise Enabler to Discover Culture Care Sunrise Model.
Source: Reprinted with permission from M. M. Leininger.

(5) *political and legal,* (6) *economic, and* (7) *educational,* forming sunrays that influence individuals, families, and groups in health and illness (Leininger, 1995a, 2002a, 2002b, 2006a). As the model indicates, it is applicable in assessing and caring for individuals, families, groups, communities, and institutions in various health systems. The CCDU theory has undergone refining for 6 decades and is used in nursing as well as in other health-related disciplines (Leininger, 1995a, 2002a; Leininger & McFarland, 2006).

Theoretical Assumptions

The formation of theoretical assumptions emanates from the major tenets of the CCDU theory (Leininger, 2006a). Three of the 11 assumptions cited by Leininger (2006a) are listed below:

- Care is the essence...and unifying focus of nursing;
- Culture care expressions, meanings, patterns...are diverse but some commonalities (universalities) exist among and between cultures;
- Every culture has generic (emic) and usually some professional (etic) care to be discovered and used for culturally congruent care practices (pp. 18–19).

Leininger (2002b) emphasizes that the nurse need not only be a mediator or broker but has to be "very knowledgeable about the client's culture and diverse factors influencing...needs and lifeways" (p. 119). Shown in constantly interacting circles, nursing care bridges generic or folk systems and professional systems—two major constructs of the CCDU. She has consistently advocated for a holistic approach in nursing care long before the term was popular. According to Leininger (2006a), the culture care theory's focus is culture and care "because they were missing...and long neglected" (p. 7) in theory development during the 1980s and 1990s.

Leininger (2002a, 2002b) places great emphasis on the role of appropriate *culturalogical* assessment when working with individuals, families, groups, and institutions to provide culturally congruent care. In the process of this assessment, the nurse "enters the client world to discover cultural knowledge that is often embedded within individual and family values" (Leininger, 2002b, p. 117). Acknowledging the time constraints in the acute settings, Leininger (2002b) suggested a short culturalogical assessment in five phases: recording of observations using all five senses; paying close attention and listening, including for generic folk practices; identification of patterns and narratives; synthesis of themes and patterns; and development of a culturally congruent care plan jointly with the client (p. 129).

The CCDU theory has three action modes for providing culturally congruent, holistic nursing care in health and well-being or when dealing with illness or dying namely *preservation and/or maintenance, accommodation and/or negotiation, and repatterning and/or restructuring* (Leininger, 2006a, p. 8). Preservation and/or maintenance refer to those decisions that maintain and preserve desirable and helpful values and beliefs. Accommodation and/or negotiation are helpful in the adaptation and transaction for care that is fitting for the culture of the individual, families, or groups. Repatterning and/or restructuring involve mutual decision-making process as the nurse modifies or changes the nursing action to achieve better health outcomes.

The Ethnonursing Method

Leininger's (1995a, 2002a, 2002b, 2006a) development of the ethnonursing method, a unique qualitative method that includes ethnography, reflects the richness of her blended preparation in nursing and anthropology. Her seminal book, *Anthropology and Nursing: Two Worlds to Blend* (1970) laid much of the groundwork of TCN. Leininger (1995) was emphatic not only in learning from the people but also in learning from them in their familiar environment. Many nurses have conducted research using the ethnonursing method, adding considerably to the body of knowledge in TCN.

Dismissing tools and instruments as "impersonal and mechanistic and fit with objectification," Leininger (2006a, p. 58) prefers to use *enablers* to denote a participatory approach and friendliness in the research process. Leininger refers to these enablers as *stranger–friend enabler* and *observation–participation–reflection enabler.* When the researcher moves from stranger (etic) to friend during the ethnonursing process, it is more possible to gather accurate and meaningful data. The model is applicable for research conducted in various settings where the nurse explores phenomena of interest (Leininger, 2006a). Basing it from anthropology, Leininger (2006a) developed the *observation–participation–reflection enabler* in the 1960s, but added *reflections* to be in keeping with the ethnonursing method. While using these enablers, this author personally experienced this during her two stays in Vietnam in the process of completing her dissertation on *The Lived Experience of Vietnamese Nurses: A Case Study* (Sagar, 2000). As the researcher moved from a newcomer to that of a friend, the Vietnamese nurses truly opened and shared stories about their journey and their struggles to "make nursing worthy as a profession in Vietnam" (Sagar, 2000, p. 168).

Analyzing data when using the ethnonursing method is a detailed rigorous process. In this way, the research will meet the criteria of "credibility, recurrent patterning, confirmability, meaning in context" (Leininger, 2006a, p. 62) and other requirements of qualitative research.

According to Leininger (2006a), there are four phases of ethnonursing analysis:

- Phase 1 entails the collection, description, and documentation of raw data;
- Phase 2 consists of identifying and categorizing "descriptors and components" (p. 62), including coding of data and studying of similarities and differences among emic and etic descriptors;
- Phase 3 involves pattern and contextual analysis whereby data are examined carefully for "saturation of ideas and patterns" (p. 62);
- Phase 4 includes synthesizing, interpreting, and analyzing for "major themes, research findings, theoretical formulations, and recommendation" (p. 62).

Leuning, Swiggum, Wiegert, and McCollough-Zander (2002) used Leininger's CCDU, along with Campinha-Bacote's (2003) culturally competent model, to develop proposed *Standards for Transcultural Nursing,* which was approved by the Transcultural Nursing Society (TCNS) in 1999. This group of two faculty academicians, and two practitioners, made up the subcommittee from the Minnesota chapter of TCNS—who spent 3 years developing what they believed will primarily foster excellence in TCN. The standards may be most beneficial in practice but may also be helpful in curriculum development, in program and hospital accreditation, and in research (Leuning et al., 2002). Again, the CCDU depicts its applicability in nursing practice, education, administration, and research.

SECTION 2. APPLICATION OF THE THEORY IN NURSING EDUCATION

"It is imperative," according to Leininger and McFarland (2002), "that transcultural nursing be explicitly taught in undergraduate and graduate programs" (p. 527). The root of this argument is the development of TCN and its profound effects in learning, teaching, and the use of evidence-based practice. Currently, the focus on cultural competence by the government, by accrediting bodies in practice (The Joint Commission [TJC], 2010), and in academia (American Association of Colleges of Nursing [AACN], 1998, 1999, 2008; National League of Nursing [NLN], 2009) are intensifying the call for formal courses in nursing programs and other health-related fields. Despite the growing evidence that graduates of nursing programs do not have the cultural competence required to care for the increasingly diverse U.S. population (Kardong-Edgreen & Campinha-Bacote, 2008), there is no standard curricular guideline or mandate as to the inclusion of knowledge, skills, and competencies needed (Lipson & Desantis, 2007; Ryan, Carlton, & Ali, 2000).

Because of its holism and systematicity, the CCDU lends itself to application in nursing education. Both Lipson and Desantis (2007) and Ryan et al. (2000) documented its adoption in graduate and undergraduate nursing programs in the United States. As the United States becomes more diverse, the CCDU will be used more frequently to guide recruitment, engaging, and retention of minority and disadvantaged nursing students.

McFarland, Mixer, Lewis, and Easley (2006) applied the culture care theory in the recruitment, engagement, and retention phases of the Opportunities for Professional Education in Nursing (OPEN) in a 3-year, federally funded project for students who were not only culturally diverse but also educationally and financially disadvantaged. This is consistent with the efforts to develop a nursing workforce that mirrors the diversity of those receiving care (Bomar & Glenn, 2004; McFarland et al., 2006; NLN, 2009; Sullivan Commission, 2004) and to eliminate disparities in health and health care as well as to promote social justice and globalization (American Nurses Association [ANA], 1991, 1995, 2003; AACN, 1998, 1999, 2008).

Few baccalaureate programs have separate transcultural courses; other programs rely on the integration of diversity and the promotion of cultural competence in nursing courses. Nursing students from diverse cultures need understanding and caring (Leininger, 1995c) as they navigate academia in their journey to completion of the nursing program. The task of preparing culturally competent nurses falls on the faculty who must educate themselves in cultural competence in order to be effective in their teaching, mentoring, and role modeling. According to Leininger (1995c), less than 20% of faculty are prepared in TCN. About 40% of baccalaureate students and 17% of master's students have had formal courses in TCN (Leininger, 1995c). In 2000, Ryan, Carlton, and Ali's survey of 610 (36% return) baccalaureate and higher programs revealed that 43% baccalaureate and 26% of master's students had formal courses in TCN. Of those reporting formal courses in TCN at the bacalaureate program, 87% have one course and 13% have several courses; at the master's level, 86% have one course and 14% have several courses (Ryan et al., 2000).

In Project OPEN, 12 out of 200 prenursing and nursing students were recruited for the qualitative evaluation. Student-focused care was used with Leininger's three modes of actions. The students found the interventions beneficial as they successfully navigated through the nursing program (McFarland et al., 2006). For example, in culture care repatterning, students were encouraged to use financial aid and decrease their working hours, thereby increasing chances of academic success.

In her nontraditional undergraduate retention and success model, Jeffreys (2004) emphasized the multiple roles nursing students play—such as parent and wage earners—in addition to pursuing nursing. Nursing education is laden with western European values and has changed slowly to reflect the values of increasingly diverse students (Jeffreys, 2004). An issue that has not received much attention is the actual racial bias in nursing textbooks. Byrne (2001) pointed out the racial bias in the portrayal of African Americans through a content analysis of three fundamentals of nursing textbooks in areas of history of nursing, cultural content, and physical assessment and hygiene. When working with these nontraditional, diverse students, Leininger's theory could be highly applicable; the characteristics of these nursing students are similar to those in the Project OPEN. Integrating concepts to promote cultural competence among educators and students will be contributing factors in student retention and in preparing a nursing workforce that is more representative of the clients being served.

The AACN (2008), with funding from the California Endowment, developed *Cultural Competency in Baccalaureate Nursing Education: End-of-Program Competencies for Baccalaureate Nursing Program Graduates and Faculty Toolkit for Integrating These Competencies into Undergraduate Curriculum.* This document, which uses Leininger's *culture care diversity and universality theory* along with four nursing models namely *Campinha-Bacote's model of cultural competence, Giger and Davidhizar's model of TCN, Purnell's model of transcultural health care, and Spector's health traditions model* (AACN, 2008), is vital in promoting cultural competence among baccalaureate nursing graduates. Leininger's textbook *Transcultural Nursing: Concepts, Theories, Research, and Practice,* in its third edition, and deemed a classic in the field (Leininger & McFarland, 2002), was instrumental in the development of TCN (Glittenberg, 2004). The textbook, along with *Culture Care Diversity and Universality: A Worldwide Nursing Theory,* second edition (Leininger & McFarland, 2006), is widely used in nursing schools. Academia has begun to embrace the field of diversity and the promotion of cultural competence (AACN,

1998, 1999, 2008; NLN, 2009)—as more and more schools offer separate courses in TCN or continue to integrate the cultural competence in nursing and related courses—recognizing its primacy as the key to reducing disparities in health care and as patients and health care providers continue to equally get more diverse.

Although the effort from the AACN and the NLN is commendable, challenges will continue in the difficult task of integrating TCN concepts in the curriculum for those schools without a formal course in cultural competence. The difficulty stems from "overloaded curriculum and the reluctance of faculty" (Leininger, 1995c, p. 14). In light of inclusion of TCN concepts in the National Council Licensure Examination (NCLEX) and in program and hospital accreditation standards, more hope is envisioned ahead. This dawning will be a tribute to Dr. Leininger whose work in TCN spans more than 6 decades. Leininger's work and those of other TCN experts constitute a remarkable body of knowledge for evidence-based practice.

While teaching Vietnamese nurse leaders from the education and administration sectors, it was apparent that respect for elders and focus on the group were important (Sagar, 2000; Sagar, 2010). The instructors of the 2-week course applied Leininger's (1995a, 2004, 2006a) preservation and maintenance mode. The instructors accomodated and negotiated as they taught nurse leaders and educators with the aid of an interpreter and translator. In repatterning and restructuring, the instructors reviewed standards from the United States and guided the nurse leaders to develop their own philosophy of nursing (Sagar, 2000). This example proves CCDU's applicability in various formal and informal educational settings. The following role play further illustrates the theory's applicability in academia.

Sample Role Play Scenario

Student A is dressed as a faculty member, wearing a suit and seated at her desk. The meeting between faculty and student is for discussion of the student's failing grade in the first exam for nursing skills. Attempting to make the student feel better, the faculty member stood up and touched the student's head.

Student B is a Vietnamese American student in a baccalaureate program. The student is dressed in low hanging denim pants and loose shirt. His head is lowered and he is avoiding eye contact; his shoulder is hunched. When his head was touched, he suddenly jerked his head.

Student C is the certified transcultural nurse. She will moderate the discussion following the role playing and will use the following questions as guide:

1. What culture care preservation and maintenance modes could the faculty use? Explain.
2. What culture care accomodation and negotiation modes could the faculty use? Explain.
3. What culture care repatterning and/or restructuring modes could the faculty use? Explain.

Instructor/Educator: Debriefing

1. Reflect on the scenario. How did you feel?
2. Discuss what you learned. What other learning needs do you have? Discuss.
3. Discuss the application of this role play in your clinical rotation.
4. Reflect on the changes needed in your own knowledge, skills, and behavior in order to incorporate culturally congruent care.

SECTION 3. APPLICATION OF THE THEORY IN NURSING PRACTICE

The United States has one of the most diverse populations in the world. In 2008, the U.S. Census Bureau predicted that the nation will further increase in racial and ethnic diversity throughout the mid-century. There is widening disparity in health care quality and access among minority populations (Agency for Healthcare Research and Quality [AHRQ], 2008) especially among African Americans, Hispanic Americans, and American Indians (Sullivan Commission, 2004). Healthy People 2020 (U.S. Department of Health and Human Services [USDHHS], 2011) has as one of its goals the elimination of these disparities. While accounting for 33% in 2000, racial or ethnic minority groups will comprise almost half of the U.S. population by the middle of this century (AHRQ, 2008; U.S. Census Bureau, 2008). Recognizing that barriers exist for diverse populations, the USDHHS Office of Minority Health developed national standards for culturally and linguistically appropriate services (CLAS) (OMH, 2001; USDHHS, 2001).

Along with CLAS and other guidelines, the Leininger's CCDU offers a structured approach to promoting culturally congruent care.

Leininger (1995b, 2002b, 2006b) warned about cultural imposition, the tendency of health care workers to impose their own belief system and values to other people or groups because of notions of superiority. This imposition may happen while providing care here in the United States or when working with developing countries in partnerships and collaborations. People have deeply ingrained cultural values and beliefs; the success of educational outreach or technological support may depend on the "applicability or fit" (Sagar, 2000) in a particular country. Leininger's CCDU (1995a, 2002a, 2006a) and sunrise model's depiction of nurses bridging generic folk practices and professional nursing is truly telling of the immense role of nurses. Furthermore, nurses are with patients 24 hours a day, 7 days a week, creating that potential for rendering culturally congruent care that enhances health care outcomes. For this reason, it is of utmost importance to promote cultural competence among all nurses (Bomar & Glenn, 2004).

Three Action Modes

Imbedded in every cultural group is a vast area of generic folk healing practices, beliefs, and traditions. Bridging generic and professional nursing care is a prerequisite to culturally congruent care (Leininger, 1995a; Leininger & McFarland, 2002, 2006). The role of a bridge is challenging and rewarding, especially the task of connecting two markedly different cultures. Wehbe-Alamah (2008), for example, showed how knowledge of traditional Muslim generic (folk) beliefs, expressions, and practices obtained from research and other sources could be integrated to professional care. Folk care included in the article pertain to caregiving, health, illness, dietary needs, privacy, modesty, death and bereavement, and other areas followed by a discussion of the use of Leininger's three modes of actions to provide culturally congruent care (Wehbe-Alamah, 2008).

Leininger's (2006a) three action modes may be used as a framework in various practice settings along with the nursing process. Employing Leininger's three action modes will call for the utmost clinical judgment and critical thinking as the nurse diagnoses, assesses, plans, implements, and evaluates care that is culturally congruent. Examining the first step of the nursing process, Munoz and Luckmann (2005) suggested revisions of some nursing diagnoses to make them culturally sensitive. One example is *noncompliance* (North American Nursing Diagnosis Association, 2005, as cited in Taylor, Lillis, LeMone, & Lynn, 2008), which needs to be modified to "non-adherence to clinical appointment schedule related to inability to access public or private transportation" (Munoz & Luckmann, 2005, p. 232). The preservation and maintenance approach may be implemented when there are generic ways that are beneficial in care. Some examples include encouraging direct care such as bathing, feeding, and other activities of daily living performed by family members who wish to directly participate in care along these areas.

Leininger's (2006a) negotiation and accomodation modes may be employed by the nurse when nursing interventions would include adaptation and negotiation with individuals and groups in order to promote culturally congruent care to promote health, prevent illness, or to cope with illness or death—for example, teaching a Filipino American patient that although garlic may lower her blood pressure, she needs to consistently take her antihypertensive medications as prescribed. The nurse also implements this mode when allowing a Muslim patient's bed to face Mecca as long as it does not interfere with another patient in a semiprivate room or with safety issues in terms of equipment hook-ups and other necessary fixtures.

When employing Leininger's (2006a) third mode, repatterning and restructuring, the nurse sets mutual decisions with the patient to use change or modification in the plan of care in order to achieve better health outcomes. For example, Table 1.1 represents the use of the repatterning/restructuring mode for a Filipino American client who is postoperative and is reluctant to take pain medication and hesitant to

TABLE 1.1 Some Repatterning/Restructuring Modes

Belief that pain is 'punishment for sins.' Patient is hesitant to take pain medication.	Nurse teaches patient about pain control; waiting too long makes pain more difficult to alleviate and control. Relief of pain may allow the patient more time for prayers to atone for sins.
Belief that advance directive is not necessary since "Death is up to God."	Nurse teaches patient about having her wishes followed when she is unable to verbalize them, her preferences honored when she no longer could verbalize them. Setting up proxy ensures that her wishes are fulfilled.

Applying Leininger's CCDU Theory to a 70-year-old Filipino American patient who is first day postoperative for right radical mastectomy.

compose a living will as well as to designate a proxy despite this being offered during admission.

As TCN becomes more and more an important area in accreditation standards, both in academia and practice, the area of certification and recertification in TCN needs revisiting and emphasis. This could further encourage nurses to learn more about TCN (Leininger, 1995a; Leininger & McFarland, 2002). Although the Certification Committee was originally established in 1988 (TCNS, 2011) there are only about 85 nurses with current certification (P. Sagar, personal communication, March 2011). Created in 2006, the Transcultural Nursing Certification Commission developed the advanced certification (CTN-A) examination for nurses with master's degrees or higher, using guidelines to make this examination on par with other specialties (TNCC Minutes, July 8, 2006) and replacing the original certification process. Presently, a task force is in the process of developing the basic certification examination (CTN-B) for implementation in 2011 (TCNS, 2011).

SECTION 4. APPLICATION OF THE THEORY IN NURSING ADMINISTRATION

The CCDU theory is needed and is quite important in nursing academic and practice administration (Leininger, 2002c, 2006b). Leininger (2006b) outlined three reasons for using the CCDU in nursing administration: shift from uniculturalism to multiculturalism, need for reexamination of organization values in recruitment and retention practices, and development of organizational structures and function consistent with cultural and gender differences in nursing. The changing demographics among patients, students, and other health care workers bring in unique needs. Truly a visionary, Leininger was way ahead of her time in predicting how TCN could impact health care and how the CCDU could be a framework in developing culturally competent care to ensure quality and equity in health care organizations.

Hubbert (2006) emphasized the vital role of TCN theoretical knowledge and skills to "guide administrators and leaders in their relationships, decisions, and skills relevant to changing organizational structures" (p. 350). The use of the CCDU presents endless possibilities in staff recruitment and retention, daily operations of clinical units, conflict management, and strategic planning. The CCDU with utilization of the ethnonursing method of research and transcultural evidence-based practice could contribute tremendously to culturally congruent care and improved outcomes of health care. There is a vast body of knowledge generated through the research of Dr. Leininger and her followers (Glittenberg, 2004; Hubbert, 2006; Leininger, 2002a, 2006b; Ryan, 2011).

A nurse administrator has the responsibility of not only promoting self-cultural competence but also making the focus of having regularly scheduled educational offerring in cultural competence for all the nursing staff. Offering continuing education (CE) hours has the advantage of providing the education component required in licensure registration, for certification or recertification and for self-development. Appendix A offers a sample CE for a workshop using Leininger's CCDU and some components of other TCN models.

Assessment of individual cultural competence has been more prevalent than organizational assessment; there is a lack of tools measuring organizational cultural competency. LaVeist, Relosa, and Sawaya (2008) conducted a validation study of the Cultural Competency Organizational Assessment (COA360), a tool for assessing and benchmarking cultural competency of health care organizations as well as its progress in managing diversity issues. The researchers invited 186 experts to rate how well COA360 questions measured CLAS standards; ratings ranged from 4.5 to 5 on a 5-point scale, equating to "well" or "very well" (LaVeist et al., 2008, p. 263).

The ANA (1991) reiterated that the interaction of provider and client involve three cultural systems namely that of the health care provider, the client, and the organization. These interactions may create conflict and barriers to health care, creating further disparities. Therefore, it behooves nursing administrators to foster cultural competence in organizational settings. Ludwig-Beymer (2008) implemented Leininger's CCDU theory to conduct an assessment of a hypothetical hospital. The CCDU provided a framework to assess the organization, which then could be compared with the values and beliefs of the groups served by the organization. Ludwig-Beymer (2008) also outlined the process of creating a culturally competent organization using assessment tools such as Leininger's (2002a, 2006a) CCDU and the forces of magnetism by the American Nurses Credentialing Center (ANCC, 2009). Ludwig-Beymer emphatically reminded us that the mandates from regulatory bodies such as TJC and accrediting groups such as the much sought-after ANCC magnet designation both require culturally competent organizations.

REFERENCES

Agency for Healthcare Research and Quality. (February, 2008). U.S. Department of Health and Human Services. *2007 National healthcare disparities report.* Rockville, MD: Author.

American Association of Colleges of Nursing. (1998). *The essentials of baccalaureate education for professional nursing practice.* Washington, DC: Author.

American Association of Colleges of Nursing. (1999). *Nursing education's agenda for the 21st century.* Washington, DC: Author

American Association of Colleges of Nursing. (2008). *Cultural competency in baccalaureate nursing education.* Washington, DC: Author.

American Nurses Association. (1991). *Position statement on cultural diversity in nursing practice.* Kansas City, MO: Author.

American Nurses Association. (1995). *Nursing's social policy statement.* Washington, DC: Author.

American Nurses Association. (2003). *Nursing's social policy statement* (2nd ed.). Washington, DC: Nurses Books.

American Nurses Credentialing Center. (2009). *Accreditation manual.* Silver Spring, MD: Author. Retrieved February 19, 2011, from http://www.nursecredentialing.org/Accreditation/ResourcesServices/2009ManualFAQ.aspx#3

Andrews, M. M. (2008). Theoretical foundations of transcultural nursing. In M. M. Andrews & J. S. Boyle (Eds.), *Transcultural concepts in nursing care* (5th ed., pp. 3–14). Philadelphia, PA: Wolters Kluwer/Lippincott Williams & Wilkins.

Bomar, P. J., & Glenn, B. J. (2004). Sociocultural influences on family health promotion and health protection. In P. J. Bomar (Ed.), *Promoting health in families: Applying family research and theory to nursing practice* (pp. 222–254). Philadelphia, PA: Elsevier.

Byrne, M. M. (2001). Uncovering racial bias in nursing fundamentals textbooks. *Journal of Nursing and Healthcare Perspectives, 22*(6), 299–303.

Campinha-Bacote, J. (2003). *The process of cultural competence in the delivery of healthcare services: A culturally competent model of care* (3rd ed.). Cincinnati, OH: Transcultural C.A.R.E. Associates.

Glittenberg, J. (2004). A transdisciplinary, transcultural model for health care. *Journal of Transcultural Nursing, 15*(1), 6–10.

Hubbert, A. (2006). Application of culture care theory for clinical nurse administrators and managers. In M. Leininger & M. McFarland (Eds.), *Culture care diversity and universality: A worldwide nursing theory* (pp. 349–364). Boston, MA: Jones & Bartlett.

Jeffreys, M. R. (2004). *Nursing student retention: Understanding the process and making a difference.* New York, NY: Springer.

Kardong-Edgreen, S., & Campinha-Bacote, J. (2008). Cultural competency of graduating US Bachelor of Science nursing students. *Contemporary Nurse, 28,* 37–44.

LaVeist, T. A., Relosa, R., & Sawaya, N. (2008). The COA360: A tool for assessing the cultural competency of healthcare organizations. *Journal of Healthcare Management, 53*(4), 257–266.

Leininger, M. M. (1970). *Anthropology and nursing: Two worlds to blend.* New York, NY: John Wiley and Sons.

Leininger, M. M. (1995a). Overview of Leininger's culture care theory. In M. M. Leininger (Ed.), *Transcultural nursing: Concepts, theories, research, and practice* (2nd ed., pp. 93–114). New York, NY: McGraw-Hill.

Leininger, M. M. (1995b). Types of health practitioners and cultural imposition. In M. Leininger (Ed.), *Transcultural nursing: Concepts, theories, research, and practice* (2nd ed., pp. 173–186). New York, NY: McGraw-Hill Companies.

Leininger, M. M. (1995c). Teaching transcultural nursing in undergraduate and graduate nursing programs. In M. Leininger (Ed.), *Transcultural nursing: Concepts, theories, research, and practice* (2nd ed., pp. 605–625). New York, NY: McGraw-Hill Companies.

Leininger, M. M. (2002a). Culture care theory: A major contribution to advance transcultural nursing knowledge and practices. *Journal of Transcultural Nursing, 13*(3), 189–192.

Leininger, M. M. (2002b). Culture care assessments for congruent competency practice. In M. Leininger & M. McFarland (Eds.), *Transcultural nursing: Concepts, theories, research, and practice* (3rd ed., pp. 117–143). New York, NY: McGraw-Hill Companies.

Leininger, M. M. (2002c). Transcultural nursing administration and consultation. In M. Leininger & M. McFarland (Eds.), *Transcultural nursing: Concepts, theories, research, and practice* (3rd ed., pp. 563–573). New York, NY: McGraw-Hill Companies.

Leininger, M. M. (2006a). Culture Care Diversity and Universality and evolution of the ethnonursing method. In M. Leininger & M. McFarland (Eds.), *Culture care diversity and universality: A worldwide nursing theory* (pp. 1–41). Sudbury, MA: Jones & Bartlett.

Leininger, M. M. (2006b). Culture care theory and uses in nursing administration. In M. Leininger & M. R. McFarland (Eds.), *Culture care diversity and universality: A worldwide nursing theory* (pp. 365–379). Sudbury, MA: Jones & Bartlett.

Leininger, M. M., & McFarland, M. R. (2002). Transcultural nursing: Curricular concepts, principles and teaching and learning activities for the 21st century. In M. Leininger & M. McFarland (Eds.), *Transcultural nursing: Concepts, theories, research, and practice* (3rd ed., pp. 527–561). New York, NY: McGraw-Hill Companies.

Leininger, M. M., & McFarland, M. (2006). *Culture care diversity and universality: A worldwide nursing theory.* Boston, MA: Jones & Bartlett.

Leuning, C. J., Swiggum, P. D., Wiegert, H. M. B., & McCollough-Zander, K. (2002). Proposed standards for transcultural nursing. *Journal of Transcultural Nursing, 13*(1), 40–46.

Lipson, J. G., & Desantis, L. A. (2007). Current approaches to integrating elements of cultural competence in nursing education. *Journal of Transcultural Nursing, 18*(1), 10S–20S.

Ludwig-Beymer, P. (2008). Creating culturally competent organizations. In M. M. Andrews & J. S. Boyle (Eds.), *Transcultural concepts in nursing* (5th ed.). Philadelphia, PA: Wolters Kluwer Health/Lippincott, Williams, & Wilkins.

McFarland, M., Mixer, S., Lewis, A. E., & Easley, C. (2006). Use of the culture care theory as a framework for the recruitment, engagement, and retention of culturally diverse nursing students in a traditionally European American baccalaureate nursing program. In M. Leininger & M. McFarland (Ed.), *Culture care diversity and universality: A worldwide nursing theory* (pp. 239–254). Boston, MA: Jones & Bartlett.

Munoz, C., & Luckmann, J. (2005). *Transcultural communication in nursing* (2nd ed.). Clifton Park, NY: Thomson Delmar Learning.

National League of Nursing. (2009). *A commitment to diversity in nursing and nursing education.* Retrieved January 26, 2011, from http://www.nln.org/aboutnln/reflection_dialogue/refl_dial_3.htm

Office of Minority Health. (2001). *Executive summary: A patient centered guide to implementing language access services in healthcare organizations.* Washington, DC: Author.

Ryan, M. (2011). A celebration of a life of commitment to transcultural nursing: Opening of the Madeleine M. Leininger Collection on Human Caring and Transcultural Nursing. *Journal of Transcultural Nursing, 22*(1), 97.

Ryan, M., Carlton, K. H., & Ali, N. (2000). Transcultural nursing concepts and experiences in nursing curricula. *Journal of Transcultural Nursing, 11*(4), 300–307.

Sagar, P. L. (2000). The lived experience of Vietnamese nurses: A case study. Ed.D. dissertation, Columbia University Teachers College, New York. Retrieved January 28, 2011, from ProQuest Dissertations & Theses (Publication No. AAT 9959348).

Sagar, P. L. (2010). Nurse educators who work in other countries: Vietnam. In J. J. Fitzpatrick, C. M. Schultz, & T. D. Aiken (Eds.), *Giving through teaching: How nurse educators are changing the world* (pp. 306–307). New York, NY: Springer.

Sullivan Commission. (2004). Missing persons: Minorities in the health professions: A Report of the Sullivan Commission on diversity in the health care workforce. Retrieved January 26, 2011, from www.jointcenter.org/healthpolicy/docs/Sullivan.pdf

The Joint Commission. (2010). Advancing effective communication, cultural competence, and patient-and family-centered care. A roadmap for hospitals. Oakbrook Terrace, IL: Author.

Transcultural Nursing Society. (2011). *Transcultural nursing certification.* Retrieved on February 19, 2011, from http://www.tcns.org/Certification.html

Taylor, C., Lillis, C., LeMone, P., & Lynn, P. (2008). *Fundamentals of nursing: The art and science of nursing care* (6th ed.). Philadelphia, PA: Lippincott, Wiliams, and Wilkins.

U.S. Census Bureau. (2008). *An older and more diverse nation by midcentury.* Retrieved November 12, 2010, from http://www.census.gov/newsroom/releases/archives/population/cb08–123.html

U.S. Department of Health and Human Services (USDHHS) Office of Minority Health. (2001). National standards on culturally and linguistically appropriate services (CLAS). Retrieved March 3, 2011 from http://minorityhealth.hhs.gov/templates/browse.aspx?lvl=2&lvlID=15

U.S. Department of Health and Human Services (USDHHS). (2011). *Healthy People 2020*. Retrieved March 3, 2011 from http://www.healthypeople.gov/2020/default.aspx

Wehbe-Alamah, H. (2008). Bridging generic and professional care practices for Muslim patients through use of Leininger's culture care modes. *Contemporary Nurse, 28*(1), 83–97.

NCLEX-TYPE TEST QUESTIONS (1–15)

1. In her theory of culture care diversity and universality (CCDU), Leininger developed which of the following research method?
A. ethnography
B. ethnonursing method
C. qualitative method
D. domain of inquiry

2. A Filipino American woman takes fresh garlic to lower her blood pressure. The nurse teaches her to take antihypertensive medication regularly. This is an example of:
A. preservation/maintenance
B. repatterning/restructuring
C. accommodation/negotiation
D. brokering

3. The nurse is caring for a postsurgical patient who believes that "pain atones for sins." The nurse reviews the plan of care with her patient, emphasizing the difficulty of pain control when an individual waits too long before taking pain medication. According to Leininger, this mode is an example of:
A. preservation/maintenance
B. repatterning/restructuring
C. accommodation/negotiation
D. culture brokering

4. The nurse systematically implements visits from family members and allows them to assist in feeding and bathing their elderly mother. This is an example of:
A. preservation/maintenance
B. repatterning/restructuring
C. accommodation/negotiation
D. brokering

5. While discussing folk medicine with an Amish client, the nurse remarked: "In the long run, Western medicine is best!" This remark is an example of:
   A. stereotyping
   B. ethnocentrism
   C. brokering
   D. racism

6. The transcultural nurse is teaching new staff nurse about Leininger's sunrise model. As she discusses the three circles of generic or folk system, nursing care, and professional system, it is important to point out that nursing care is the:
   A. division between generic and professional systems
   B. collaboration between generic and professional systems
   C. demarcation between generic and professional systems
   D. bridge between generic and professional systems

7. The nurse moved the Muslim patient's bed so he could face east to Mecca when he prays. This is an example of:
   A. preservation/maintenance
   B. repatterning/restructuring
   C. accommodation/negotiation
   D. brokering

8. The nurse knocks on the door and pauses prior to entering the door of a female Muslim client to give the client time to cover her head. This is an example of:
   A. accommodation/negotiation
   B. preservation/maintenance
   C. repatterning/restructuring
   D. brokering

9. According to Leininger, health care workers may have a tendency for notion of superioriy and may impose their own belief system when working here or abroad. This process is referred to as:
   A. accommodation/negotiation
   B. repatterning/restructuring
   C. cultural brokering
   D. cultural imposition

10. The nurse educator encourages her academic advisee to use more financial aid and work less hours to be able to devote more time studying. This is an example of:
    A. accommodation/negotiation
    B. preservation/maintenance
    C. repatterning/restructuring
    D. brokering

11. The nurse supervisor approves a 4-week vacation for a staff nurse from India requesting 6 weeks vacation to care of a sick relative at home. This is an example of:
    A. accommodation/negotiation
    B. preservation/maintenance
    C. repatterning/restructuring
    D. brokering

12. The Leininger CCDU theory is illustrated as the sunrise model to depict:
    A. hope to generate new ways of knowing in nursing
    B. hope to generate more theory in nursing
    C. hope to generate new knowledge in nursing
    D. hope to generate more caring in nursing

13. The Leininger CCDU theory is focused on culture and care. According to Leininger, culture and care:
    A. were the focus in theory development during the 1980s and 1990s
    B. were long neglected and missing in theory development during the 1980s and 1990s
    C. were returning in theory development during the 1980s and 1990s
    D. were the trend in theory development during the 1980s and 1990s

14. Leininger cited which of the following as the cause for the difficulty in integrating transcultural concepts in nursing curricula?
    A. overloaded curriculum and reluctance of faculty
    B. overloaded curriculum and indifference of faculty
    C. overloaded curriculum and refusal of faculty
    D. overloaded curriculum and lack of motivation of faculty

15. Leininger acknowledges which of the following concepts within and between cultures?
A. similarities only
B. differences only
C. similarities and differences
D. comparison only

(Answers to these questions can be found on p. 143)

2

LARRY PURNELL'S MODEL FOR CULTURAL COMPETENCE

SECTION 1. REVIEW OF THE MODEL

The Purnell model for cultural competence (PMCC), developed in 1991, was initially a framework for clinical assessment tool (Purnell, 2002). Dr. Larry Purnell's book, *Culturally Competent Health Care*, won the 2006 American Journal of Nursing Award while his other book *Transcultural Health Care: A Culturally Competent Approach* is the recipient of the Brandon Hill Book Award (Purnell, 2007). Purnell coauthored *Developing Cultural Competence in Physical Therapy* with Lattanzi; this book was adopted by the Center for International Rehabilitation and Research Information Exchange (Purnell, 2007). The Commission on Internationalization and Cultural Competence for the European Union project for the Bologna-Sorbonne-Salamanca World Health Organization declarations has retained Dr. Purnell as consultant and has adopted the PMCC as framework (Purnell, 2007).

The PMCC shows a circle with four rims: (1) global society (ouside rim); (2) community (second rim); (3) family (third rim); and (4) individual (fourth rim) (Purnell, 2002, 2004, 2005, 2008) (Figure 2.1). The dark center of the circle denotes the unknown.

Purnell (2002, 2008) used a jagged line on the bottom of the circle to illustrate the "nonlinear concept of cultural competence" (p. 20). Furthermore, Purnell (2008) listed four levels of cultural competence, namely, *unconsciously incompetent, consciously incompetent, consciously competent, and unconsciously competent* (p. 21). Unconsciously incompetent is defined as the absence of awareness that one lacks knowledge

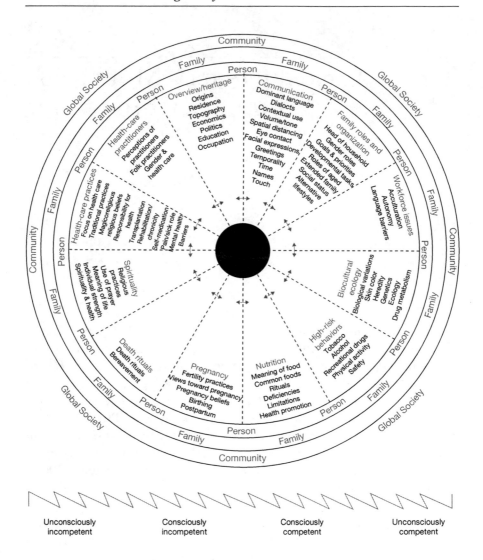

Primary characteristics of culture: age, generation, nationality, race, color, gender, religion

Secondary characteristics of culture: educational status, socioeconomic status, occupation, military status, political beliefs, urban versus rural residence, enclave identity, marital status, parental status, physical characteristics, sexual orientation, gender issues, and reason for migration (sojourner, immigrant, undocumented status)

Unconsciously incompetent: not being aware that one is lacking knowledge about another culture
Consciously incompetent: being aware that one is lacking knowledge about another culture
Consciously competent: learning about the client's culture, verifying generalizations about the client's culture, and providing culturally specific interventions
Unconsciously competent: automatically providing culturally congruent care to clients of diverse cultures

FIGURE 2.1 Purnell's model for cultural competence.
Source: Reprinted with permission from Larry D. Purnell, PhD, RN, FAAN.

about other cultures; consciously incompetent denotes presence of awareness about the lack of that knowledge; consciously competent describes learning about the client's culture and rendering culturally fit interventions; and unconsciously competent refers to the innate provision of culturally congruent care to multicultural clients (Purnell, 2008). The four rims, along with conscious competence, make up the macrolevel of the PMCC.

The PMCC aims to provide a framework for all health care providers to study cultural concepts and characteristics and to interrelate characteristics of culture to promote culturally competent and sensitive health care (Purnell, 2008). According to Purnell (2008), there are 20 assumptions that serve as basis for the PMCC; three of the 20 assumptions are as follows:

- Culture has a powerful influence on one's interpretation of and responses to health care;
- Caregivers need both culture-general and culture-specific information in order to provide culturally . . . competent care;
- Caregivers who can assess, plan, intervene, and evaluate in a culturally competent manner will improve the care of clients whom they serve (p. 20).

Cultural Domains

Twelve pie-like wedges reflecting cultural *domains* are within the circle of the PMCC. The 12 domains or *constructs* furnish the organizing framework of the model; these interconnecting domains could be used as a guide in patient assessment in diverse care settings (Purnell, 2002, 2008). According to Purnell (2002, 2004, 2008), the 12 domains comprise the microlevel of the model. The broken lines between the 12 domains show the interconnectedness of the model (American Association of Colleges of Nursing [AACN], 2008; Purnell, 2002, 2008).

The first domain is "overview, inhabited localities, and topography" (Purnell, 2008, pp. 22–23). These interrelated concepts inlude the person's native land, present residence, health, economics, migration, and educational level, among others. These concepts affect each other and have direct bearing in migration, responses to health and illness, and access and quality of care.

Purnell (2008) acknowledges that the second domain, "communication" (pp. 27–30), is the most complex-inclusive of verbal language skills as well as nonverbal aspects such as eye contact, touch, appropriate greetings, and time orientation. Thirdly, "family roles and organizations" is the relationships between those who are inside and outside and encompass gender roles, roles for elderly and extended family members, and sanctions for alternate lifestyles (Purnell, 2008, pp. 30–33).

Purnell (2008) cites "workforce issues" (pp. 33–36) as the fourth cultural domain and focuses on language barriers, acculturation, and autonomy. Evidence of minority representation in nursing is glaring. According to the American Nurses Association in 2006, there are only 4.2% African Americans, 3.4% Asian/Pacific Islanders, 1.6% Hispanic/Latinos, and 0.4% Native Americans out of all nurses in the United States (as cited by Purnell, 2008). The Sullivan Commission (2004) reported that while African American, Hispanic Americans, and American Indians constitute 25% of the U.S. population, there are less than 10% nurses from those three ethnic groups. In times of cyclical nursing shortages, health care facilities in the United States have employed nurses from developing countries such as the Philippines, India, and China and from developed nations such as Canada and England.

The fifth domain is "biocultural ecology" comprising the physical, biologic, and physiologic differences among ethnic and racial groups (Purnell, 2008, pp. 36–40). Purnell (2008) cites "high-risk behaviors" as the sixth domain; this consists of tobacco and other drug use; sedentary lifestyle; and risks associated with recreational drugs, unsafe driving, and sexually transmitted diseases (pp. 38–40). "Nutrition" accounts for the seventh domain including meaning of food; its associated rituals, deficiences in intake; and role in promoting health and wellness, preventing illness, and restoring health (Purnell, 2008).

The eigth domain is "pregnancy and childbearing practices"; under this domain are culturally approved means of fertility, pregnancy, birth, and postpartum rituals (Purnell, 2008, pp. 43–44). Purnell's (2008) ninth cultural domain is "death rituals" inclusive of views about death and dying—rituals for death, burial, and mourning.

Purnell (2008) emphasized that the domain of "spirituality" includes not only religious beliefs but also its encompassing effects on other cultural domains particularly nutrition and health practices. The eleventh domain consists of "health care practices" that cover traditional beliefs and practices; views about individual health, mental illness, organ donation; and manifestations of pain and of being ill (Purnell, 2008). The last domain "health care practitioners" covers the perception about and use of health care providers (Purnell, 2005,

2008). The PMCC is eclectic and conceptualizes many theories with each domain affecting and affected by the other domains. According to Purnell (2002), cultural competence is not linear and is the "adaptation of care in a manner that is consistent with the culture of the client..." (p. 193). Purnell (2001) warns against borderline cultural imposition practices such as ordering a specific diet while disregarding cultural preferences or allowing only immediate family to visit the client.

The AACN (2008) chose Purnell's model of transcultural health care along with the theory by Leininger and models by Campinha-Bacote; Giger and Davidhizar; and Spector to develop the *Cultural Competency in Baccalaureate Nursing Education* (AACN, 2008). This document provides a framework for the inclusion of cultural competence in baccalaureate nursing curricula.

While they could not ascertain how many and which schools use what model, Lipson and Desantis (2007) noted that the Purnell model is one of the most widely used in nursing school curricula. Like Giger and Davidhizar, Purnell organizes his book around ethnic and immigrant groups. The model has applicability in practice, education, administration, and research in nursing and other health-related fields; it has been used worldwide, necessitating translation into Flemish, French, Korean, Spanish (Purnell, 2002), Portuguese, and Turkish (Purnell, 2007).

SECTION 2. APPLICATION OF THE MODEL IN NURSING EDUCATION

The PMCC can be applied to different levels of nursing education. Purnell's (2002, 2004, 2008) 12 domains of culture may easily be threaded into the theoretical nursing courses and in clinical experiences. The domains could be used as assessment parameters; this could be woven into the physical assessment course as a guiding framework or as a tool to be used as an adjunct to the nursing process in the care of assigned clients in all clinical courses. Assessing and planning care with the use of the 12 cultural domains may be a tool to ensure that cultural diversity and promotion of cultural competence are integrated into nursing curricula. In addition to nurses, nutritionists, physicians, physical therapists, anthropologists, and social workers use the PMCC not only in academia but also in staff development settings (Purnell, 2007). Because of its simplicity, it could be used in beginning nursing

TABLE 2.1 Weaving Purnell's 12 Domains Into the Weekly Assessment Tool for an Adult Health Nursing Course

Sample Weekly Assignment: NUR 300–Adult Health Nursing
Student: Date:
Patient's Initials: RT   Age: 23   Sex: F   Marital Status: Married   Religion: Roman Catholic
Admission Date: 12/12/10   Medical Dx: Uncontrolled Diabetes Mellitus; Pregnancy, 8 Weeks.

Domain	Assessment	Plan	Rationale
Overview, inhabited localities, topography	"I came to this country 7 years ago. No, no citizen. Just working."	1. Assess level of education.	1. Will influence teaching methods and materials.
Communication	Looks down frequently when speaking with nurses. "I learned English working at a convent in Tijuana."	1. Accept and respect this communication pattern.	1. Respect is of prime importance among Mexican Americans.
Family roles and organizations	"My husband works as a gardener but jobs are difficult to find. I clean houses, get money off the books."	1. Respect concept of familism. 2. Emphasize confidentiality. 3. Accommodate visit with extended family in a systematic manner (rotation).	1. An encompassing value among Mexican Americans. 2. Will foster trust in the health care worker. 3. Extended family is important.
Biocultural ecology	Black haired and dark-skinned. Weighs 200 lbs., 5 feet height. "I no go for immunizations. I bring kids for shots. My husband? No go."	1. Assess for cyanosis at buccal mucosa, tongue, lips; for jaundice, check conjuntivae and buccal mucosa. 2. Teach preventive measures against chemical cleaning agents, pesticide, communicable diseases.	1. Will offer more accurate parameters among dark-skinned peoples. 2. Many Mexicans use these in work settings and live in crowded housing situations.
High risk behaviors	"I no drink alcohol; just beer on weekends when family get together. Yes, me and my husband smoke.One half pack for me. A pack for him."	1. Teach about alcohol content of beer and other beverages. Relate to DM and its effect on the unborn baby. 2. Teach effects of nicotine to both smokers, unborn baby, and passive smokers. Relate to DM and pregnant status.	1. And 2. These interventions may help in reducing alcohol intake and smoking during pregnancy. It may also prevent husband from smoking in the house.

Category	Data	Interventions
Nutrition	Weighs 200 lbs., 5 feet height. "No walking. My feet hurts when I walk. When no hurting, no time to walk. My son goes to school; the baby stays with my mother."	1. Assess use of hot and cold practices in terms of food and illnesses. 2. Find our usual food at mealtimes, preparation methods, as well as portions.
Pregnancy and chidbearing practices	" Got 2 sons, seven and 2 year old. The older go to school. Sometime he take care of the baby when my mother work cleaning houses, too." "I no go for check-up yet (touches abdomen). I go when I get more money to pay."	1. Refer to free clinic for prenatal care. 2. Teach dangers of prenatal care to self and baby
Death rituals	"I no hear about advanced directives." "I no believe in organ donation."	1. Allow verbalizations of beliefs about health and illness, treatment. 2. Respect patients beliefs and decisions. 3. Give information about Patient Self-Determination Act.
Spirituality	Wearing a crucifx pinned to hospital gown. A rosary and a small picture of the Virgin Mary sits atop the bedside table. " I go to mass with my family when no work on Sundays."	1. Allow verbalizations about soul or spirit. 2. Respect and allow space for this altar 3. Assess need to speak with the priest or receive communion.
Health care practices	Has no health insurance. "I first go to curandero when I'm sick"	1. Assess use of traditional practitioners
Health care practitioners	Appears hesitant to share information	1. Treat with respect 2. Emphasize confidentiality 3. Inquire about the health of other family members

And in the rightmost column (rationale):

Nutrition:
1. Many Mexian Americans use hot and cold balance to restore bodily harmony.
2. Will assist in planning teaching.

Spirituality:
1. Most Mexicans enjoy talking about this especially in times of illness.
2. Shows respect for client and her religious practices.

Health care practices:
1. Avoid conflicting treatment.

Health care practitioners:
1. Respect is of prime importance
2. Will build trust; dispel fear of disclosure about undocumented status.
3. The family is of prime importance among Mexican Americans

Source: Developed using Purnell, L. D. (2008). The Purnell Model for cultural competence In L. D. Purnel & B. J. Paulanka (Eds.), Transcultural health care: A culturally competent approach (3rd ed., pp. 19–55) and Zoucha, R., & Zamarripa, C. A. (2003). People of Mexian heritage. In L. D. Purnell & B. J. Paulanka (Eds.), Transcultural health care: A culturally competent approach (3rd ed., pp. 309–324). Philadelphia, PA: FA Davis.

classes and in short transcultural immersion courses here and abroad (Purnell, 2007).

To explore teaching and learning methods involved incorporating cultural competence in the curricula, Lipson and Desantis (2007) conducted a survey of schools by telephone, electronic mail, and face–face interviews. Their findings indicate that knowledge, attitudes, and skills in cultural competence are included in nursing programs through (1) specialty focus, (2) required courses, (3) models, (4) immersion experiences, and (5) distance learning or simulation (Lipson & Desantis, 2007). Specialties at the master's level may comprise three or more courses in cultural competence in addition to other program requirements. In some schools, required nursing courses may vary: "transcultural nursing, cross-cultural nursing…health and culture, diversity…health disparities" (Lipson & Desantis, 2007, p. 12S). Lipson and Desantis concluded that some schools use the following theory by Leininger and models by Purnell, Campinha-Bacote, Giger, and Davidhizar while other programs develop courses around books such as those of Andrews and Boyle and Spector; yet it is difficult to determine the actual number of schools and the models used. Table 2.1 weaves Purnell's 12 domains into the weekly assessment tool for an Adult Health Nursing Course.

SECTION 3. APPLICATION OF THE MODEL IN NURSING PRACTICE

Purnell (2008) views cultural competence as a journey; at play in this journey are the willingness and capacity of an individual to provide culturally congruent care to clients. On this journey, Purnell (2008) provides general guidelines that include openness to learning other cultures; willingness to work with clients of diverse cultures; and being responsible for own development of cultural competence through reading, conferences, and accessing learning materials. The above assessment tool—appying PMCC to nursing education and care planning guide—is applicable to use in various clinical settings. Nurses, physicians, physical therapists, and social workers in the United States, Canada, Central America, and Europe use the PMCC for clients in acute, long-term, and home care settings (Purnell, 2007). According to Purnell (2007), another notable use of the PMCC is the adoption by the Oncology Nursing Society in developing its standards and its selection and placement by a New Jersey hospital of various chapters of *Transcultural Health Care: A Culturally Competent Approach* into their intranet.

Another use of the model is in community health nursing. For example, the nurse providing primary care in all three levels of prevention could focus in the domain of communication with other clients and health care workers.When communicating, the nurse must be sensitive to verbal and nonverbal means of communication, taking care to maintain respect and culturally congruent practices in all encounters. A medical interpreter must be available either as part of the team or by accessing the language access services. All other cultural domains could be applied here as well.

Continuing and mandatory education programs need to address diversity and promotion of cultural competence (Purnell, 2008). In such programs, general topics in culture and those specific to clientele being served must be included. Furthermore, Purnell (2008) emphasized that cultural resourses must be available for the staff in-unit and in the library; that nurses, pharmacists, and physicians must receive continuing education in ethnopharmacology; and that mentoring programs be available to the staff.

In addition, Purnell (2008) suggested certification in transcultural nursing in both advanced (CTN-A) and basic (CTN-B) levels must be available and promoted among the staff nurses. Recognition for certified staff, whether in staff honor roll or with monetary incentive diferential or both, will boost morale and add to the value of certification. Unlike other certifications, the CTN has not received its due recognition and prestige. It has been 2 years since the Transcultural Nursing Certification Commission had developed the revised certification exam but many hospitals and schools of nursing are still not aware of its existence (P. L. Sagar, personal communication, January 20, 2011).

In consonance with Healthy People 2020 (U.S. Department of Health and Human Services [USDHHS], 2011), cultural domains from the PMCC including communication, risk factors for diseases, health care practices, nutrition, among others (Purnell, 2004, 2008), may be used to plan health promotion sessions such as smoking cessation, avoidance of alcohol, prevention of human immune deficiency/ acquired immune deficiency syndrome. Table 2.2 outlines levels of prevention for individuals at a migrant community.

When using evidence-based practice, Purnell (2008) strongly advocated for more research dealing with efficacy of interventions or care preference by cultural groups. General culture and culture-specific knowledge—he reiterated—guide clinicians to be more client focused in assessing, planning, providing, and evaluating culturally congruent care (Purnell, 2008).

TABLE 2.2 Outlines Levels of Prevention for Individuals at a Migrant Community

Level of Prevention	Activities	Domains of Culture According to Purnell
Primary	1. Conduct teaching sessions about reduction of exposure to pesticides 2. Teach about tuberculosis, its signs and symptoms, treatment, and prevention of transmission	1. And 2. Biocultural ecology, high risk behavior, overview and heritage
Secondary	Provide screening activities during a health fair such as urine testing for pesticide exposure	Biocultural ecology, high risk behavior, overview and heritage
Tertiary	1. Refer for treatment of skin irritations, nausea and vomiting 2. Teach those receiving treatment for TB to complete treatment	Biocultural ecology, high risk behavior, overview and heritage.

Source: Developed from Bushy, A., & Napolitano, M. (2010). Rural Health and migrant health. In M. Stanhope and J. Lancaster *Foundations of nursing in the community: Community-oriented practice* (3rd ed.). St. Louis, MO: Elsevier Mosby and from Purnell, L. D. (2008). *Transcultural health care: A culturally competent approach.* Philadelphia, PA: FA Davis.

Nieto-Vasquez, Tejeda, Colin, and Matos (2009) conducted a study to determine the effects of an osteoporosis educational intervention on knowledge, health beliefs, and efficacy among 105 Puerto Rican women in college. The researchers used four of Purnell's 12 cultural domains: biocultural ecology, high-risk behavior, nutrition, and health care practices. The educational intervention was in Spanish and was developed both from the guidelines of the National Osteoporosis Foundation for Women and from consultation with an expert in Puerto Rican culture as well as osteoporosis (Nieto-Vazquez et al., 2009). Findings indicated that the experimental group had significantly more knowledge and positive beliefs than the control group. This study shows the applicability of the PMCC in practice and research and how selected domains could be used as theoretical framework.

In a case study involving the creation of a Web site on *Cultural Competency and Haitian Immigrants* for public health personnel in rural Delaware, Phelps and Johnson (2004) succeeded in showing another application of the PMCC in practice. The project coordinators selected the PMCC because of its "comprehensiveness and application to many disciplines…"(Phelps & Johnson, 2004, p. 208). Unlike Nieto-Vazquez et al. (2009) who used only four of the cultural domains, these researchers used all 12 domains of the PMCC. In this age of technological breakthrough, the availability of quality and user friendly online resources will assist health care professionals and clients (Cater, 2009); this is consistent with

Healthy People 2010 and the proposed Healthy People 2020 objectives (USDHHS, 2000, 2011). Specifically, this is a more accessible strategy for health care workers—who may have difficulty attending face to face conferences—in their respective journeys to cultural competence. For project continuity and usefulness, Phelps and Johnson (2004) suggested the maintenance of the Web site in terms of currency of information, the provision of further links to Haitian resources, and the evaluation of site use by health care workers. The electronic delivery of staff development education in this project opens the possibilities of other use of the PMCC.

SECTION 4. APPLICATION OF THE MODEL IN NURSING ADMINISTRATION

Purnell (2008) is emphatic in saying that individual competence is not enough; the institution delivering care must also make evident its commitment to cultural competence. The PMCC could be used in nurse administration settings along with Culturally and Linguistically Appropriate Services (CLAS) (USDHHS, Office of Minority Health, 2001) and The Joint Commission (2010a, 2010b) guidelines. Just like individual competence, the process of organizational competence is also a journey.

Administrators have used the PMCC and its organizing framework in cross-cultural and multinational populations among health care professionals (Purnell, 2007). The PMCC is used in care planning for specifc cultural populations in long-term care settings and in ethics committees' assessment of clients' adherence to care and appropriateness of care from both staff and client perspectives (Purnell, 2007).

According to Purnell et al. (2011), an organization must first asses its strengths, weaknesses, and capacities in four key components: (1) administration and governance; (2) orientation and education; (3) language services; and (4) staff competencies. An inclusive board of governance needs a member of the ethnicity of the community being served. Orientation and education activities must include all levels of the organization from the chief executive officer to housekeeping (Purnell et al., 2011). Language, the third component, has been cited as the biggest barrier to health care (USDHHS, OMH, 2001) especially in a country where most health care providers assume that everyone can read, write, and understand English and most patient assessment and education tools are in English. The CLAS standards, a set of mandates and guidelines, are key to planning for development of staff knowledge, skill, and competencies. Workshops with continuing education credits on culturally congruent care for the ethnic groups served, on ethnopharmacology, and on information literacy, are important areas for staff competencies. While individuals must be responsible for their continuing education, Purnell et al. (2011) recommend encouragement and provision of financial resources and time to attend educational conferences.

The nurse administrator will need to collaborate with nurse educators from staff development to include Purnell's (2002, 2004, 2008) cultural domains and may use the 12 domains or selected domains of culture, for example, when planning for orientation of new staff members. Purnell (2004) advocates for the inclusion of cultural aspects in terms of assessment tool for client admission and those that are vital and used frequently such as a pain assessment tool in the language of the clients served. Purnell (2008, 2011) also suggested the formation of a *Cultural Competence Committee* composed of staff and administrators, clergy, and community representatives. This composition is similar to hospitals and other institutions' ethics committee.

REFERENCES

American Association of Colleges of Nursing. (2008). *Cultural competency in baccalaureate nursing education.* Washington, DC: Author.

Bushy, A., & Napolitano, M. (2010). Rural health and migrant health. In M. Stanhope & J. Lancaster (Eds.), *Foundations of nursing in the community: Community-oriented practice* (3rd ed., pp. 400–418). St. Louis, MO: Elsevier Mosby.

Cater, K. C. (2009). Informatics and technology in professional nursing practice. In K. Masters (Ed.), *Role development in professional nursing practice* (2nd ed., pp. 287–300). Sudbury, MA: Jones & Bartlett.

Lipson, J. G., & Desantis, L. A. (2007). Current approaches to integrating elements of cultural competence in nursing education. *Journal of Transcultural Nursing, 18*(1), 10S–20S.

Nieto-Vasquez, M. N., Tejeda, M. J., Colin, J., and Matos, A. M. (2009). Results of an osteoporosis educational intervention randomized trial in a sample of Puerto-Rican women. *Journal of Cultural Diversity, 16*(4), 171–177.

Office of Minority Health. (2001). Executive summary: A patient centered guide to implementing language access services in healthcare organizations. Washington, DC: Author.

Phelps, L. D., & Johnson, K. (2004). Developing local public health capacity in cultural competency: A case study with Haitians in a rural community. *Journal of Community Health Nursing, 21*(4), 203–215.

Purnell, L. D. (2001). Cultural competence in a changing health care environment. In N. L. Chaska (Ed)., *The nursing profession: Tomorrow and beyond* (pp. 451–460). Thousand Oaks, CA: Sage.

Purnell, L. D. (2002). The Purnell model for cultural competence. *Journal of Transcultural Nursing, 13*(3), 193–196.

Purnell, L. D. (2004). *Guide to culturally competent care* (2nd ed.). Philadelphia, PA: FA Davis.

Purnell, L. D. (2005). The Purnell model for cultural competence. *Journal of Multicultural Nursing & Health, 11*(2), 7–15.

Purnell, L. D. (2007). Comentary on "Current approaches to integrating elements of cultural competence in nursing education." *Journal of Transcultural Nursing, 18*(1), 23S–24S.

Purnell, L. D. (2008). The Purnell model for cultural competence. In L. D. Purnel & B. J. Paulanka. *Transcultural health care: A culturally competent approach* (3rd ed., pp. 19–55). Philadelphia, PA: FA Davis.

Purnell, L. D., Davidhizar, R. E., Giger, J. N., Strickland, O. L., Fishman, D., & Allison, D. M. (2011). A guide to developing culturally competent organizations. *Journal of Transcultural Nursing, 22*(1), 7–14.

Sullivan Commission. (2004). *Missing persons: Minorities in the health professions: A report of the Sullivan Commission on diversity in the health care workforce.* Retrieved January 26, 2011, from http://www.jointcenter.org/healthpolicy/docs/Sullivan.pdf

The Joint Commission. (2010a). *Advancing effective communication, cultural competence, and patient- and family-centered care: A roadmap for hospitals.* Oakbrook Terrace, IL: Author.

The Joint Commission. (2010b). *Cultural and linguistic care in area hospitals.* Oakbrook Terrace, IL: Author.

U.S. Department of Health and Human Services, Office of Minority Health. (2001). *Culturally and linguistically appropriate services.* Retrieved August 26, 2010, from http://www.usdhhs.gov

U.S. Department of Health and Human Services. (2010). *Healthy People 2020.* Accessed 12 January, 2011, from http://www.healthypeople.gov/HP2020/Objectives/selectionCriteria.aspx

U.S. Department of Health and Human Services. (2000). *Healthy People 2020.* Accessed 12 January, 2011, from http://www.healthypeople.gov/2010/LHI/lhiwhat.htm

Zoucha, R., & Zamarripa, C. A. (2008). People of Mexican heritage. In L. D. Purnell, & B. J. Paulanka (Eds.), *Transcultural health care: A culturally competent approach* (3rd ed., pp. 309–324). Philadelphia, PA: FA Davis.

NCLEX-TYPE TEST QUESTIONS (1–15)

1. The nurse is planning care to increase activity for a 25-year-old Mexican American client. Which of the following activities would the client be more likely to do?
   A. dancing for at least 30 minutes 3 to 4 times a week
   B. walking for at least 30 minutes 4 times a week
   C. exercising in the gym at least 30 minutes 4 times a week
   D. playing golf at least 30 minutes 4 times a week

2. The Purnell model for cultural competence has four rims. Which rim represents the person?
   A. inner
   B. first
   C. second
   D. third

3. While communicating with her Japanese American client, the nurse notices that the client is avoiding eye contact. This manifestation of nonverbal communication is a sign of:
   A. acculturation to the dominant culture
   B. respect for authority
   C. disinterest in the nurse
   D. inattentiveness to the nurse

4. The transcultural nurse is providing orientation to a group of new nurses. Which of the following would be the nurse's best explanation for the language access services?
   A. "The language access services is provided for patients who are unable to speak English and for those who have limited English proficiency."
   B. "The language access services is provided with nominal charge for patients who are unable to speak English and for those who have limited English proficiency."
   C. "The language access services is provided free of charge for patients who are unable to speak English only."
   D. "The language access services is provided free of charge for patients who are unable to speak English and for those who have limited English proficiency."

5. A newly diagnosed Jewish diabetic patient who has been pre-scribed Humulin insulin exclaimed: "I will not be able to take insu-lin because of religious reasons!" Which of the following replies by the nurse is most accurate?
   A. "Humulin is pork insulin derived from recombinant DNA technology."
   B. "Humulin is beef insulin derived from recombinant DNA technology."
   C. "Humulin is human insulin derived from recombinant DNA technology."
   D. "Humulin is sheep insulin derived from recombinant DNA technology."

6. Which of the following food items would be contraindicated in a full liquid diet for a strictly vegetarian patient?
   A. vegetable broth
   B. jello
   C. tea
   D. ginger ale

7. Your Muslim client is very concerned and is requesting you to find out the ingredients in one of his medications in gelatin capsule form. You suspect that the client is concerned that the gelatin is made up of:
   A. pork derivative
   B. chicken derivative
   C. beef derivative
   D. turkey derivative

8. The jagged lines below the circle in Purnell's model represents the:
   A. linear concept of cultural consciousness
   B. semilinear concept of cultural consciousness
   C. nonlinear concept of cultural consciousness
   D. unknown concept of cultural consciousness

9. Purnell recommends that nurses, physicians, and pharmacists learn ethnopharmacology. The main reason for this suggestion is:
   A. the wide variations in drug metabolism among racial and ethnic groups
   B. the small variations in drug metabolism among racial and ethnic groups

    C. the specific alterations in drug metabolism among racial and ethnic groups

    D. the nonspecifc variations in drug metabolism among racial and ethnic groups

10. According to Purnell, the topography of a given country or region may provide the health care practitioners with:
    A. essential clues to symptoms requiring investigation
    B. knowledge of risk factors to enhance the diagnostic process
    C. knowledge of new and reemerging illnesses
    D. symptoms of specific illnesses

11. The nurse caring for a Chinese American client with kidney stones observed that the iced water on the bedside table is untouched despite her explanations to force fluid. Which of the following would be the most therapeutic response by the nurse?
    A. "I see that you have not drank any of the iced water. The doctor will be upset."
    B. "I see that you have not drank any of the iced water. You will have more difficulty passing the stones."
    C. "I see that you have not drank any of the iced water. Would you like some cranberry juice?"
    D. "I see that you have not drank any of the iced water. Is there any other fluid you would prefer?"

12. A hospital working on magnet status application has hired a certified transcultural nurse with advanced certification (CTN-A) to lead its staff development program. Which of the following approaches by the CTN would be most helpful in the beginning attempt to ensure the hospital's compliance with Culturally and Linguistically Appropriate Services standards?
    A. Determine if hospital receives state funding and if language access services is in place.
    B. Determine if hospital receives federal funding and if language access services is in place.
    C. Determine if hospital receives private funding and if language access services is in place.
    D. Determine if hospital is nonprofit and if language access services are in place.

13. The father of a new born baby refused the invitation to see mother and baby immediately after birth. Which of the following responses by the nurse would be most culturally sensitive?
    A. "Most fathers would like to see the baby after birth."
    B. "Please let us know when it is best for you to see the baby."
    C. "Most fathers prefer to stay with the mother during delivery."
    D. "When you are ready, please let us know."

14. While teaching physical assessment in the skills laboratory, the clinical instructor explains techniques for assessment of dark-skinned clients' oxygenation wherein the practitioner must examine the client's:
    A. buccal mucosa, tongue, lips
    B. earlobes, tongue, lips
    C. hands, feet, buccal mucosa
    D. forehead, tongue, lips

15. The client stated that he sees a folk healer prior to consulting with a health care practitioner. This practice is an example of Purnell's cultural domain of:
    A. high-risk behavior
    B. overview and topography
    C. workforce issues
    D. health care practices

    (Answers to these questions can be found on p. 144)

3

JOSEPHA CAMPINHA-BACOTE'S
THE PROCESS OF CULTURAL COMPETENCE IN THE DELIVERY OF HEALTHCARE SERVICES AND *BIBLICALLY BASED MODEL OF CULTURAL COMPETENCE*

SECTION 1. REVIEW OF THE MODEL

Dr. Josepha Campinha-Bacote (2007) started developing the first version of *The Process of Cultural Competence in the Delivery of Healthcare Services* in 1991 with four constructs: *cultural awareness, cultural knowledge, cultural skill,* and *cultural encounters* (p. 17). The model blended the work of Leininger in 1978 and Pedersen in 1988 (Campinha-Bacote, 2002). In 2003, she further integrated the works of Kleinman in 1978 and Law in 1993 while in 2005 she added the works of Chapman into the model (Campinha-Bacote, 2007). To create the representation of her model, Campinha-Bacote (2007) showed four interconnected concepts of cultural awareness, cultural knowledge, cultural skill, and cultural encounter standing on a base labeled "cultural competence" (p. 17).

This first version's graphic representation of *The Process of Cultural Competence in the Delivery of Healthcare Services* model could be accesesed on the Transcultural Clinical Administrative Research and Education (C.A.R.E.) Web site at http://www.transculturalcare.net, a private organization that provides presentations, workshops, and consultation conducted by Dr. Josepha Campinha-Bacote. Campinha-Bacote's model was used (along with Leininger's culture care diversity

and universality theory) by Leuning et al. (2002) to create the standards
for transcultural nursing (TCN).

Evolution of the Model

Cultural knowledge consists of having a solid foundation regarding diverse cultures; this process of actively seeking sound basis
enables the health care professional to understand different worldviews (Campinha-Bacote, 2003a, 2007). Resources in obtaining this
knowledge include textbooks, computer programs, literary works,
and spiritual sources. The person's worldview influences responses
to health, illness, or disability. *Cultural encounters* involve face-to-face
cultural interactions with diverse clients to validate or clarify beliefs
about those groups (Campinha-Bacote, 2003a, 2007). Culturally skillful practitioners are not only able to collect pertinent data about the
client but also proficient in culturally appropriate physical examination. Various tools and guides available for the purpose of physical examination include those of Leininger (2002, 2006a), Giger and
Davidhizar (2008), Purnell (2008), Spector (2009), and Andrews and
Boyle (2008).

To dispel the notion of the linearity of the process of cultural
competence, Campinha-Bacote (2003a, 2011) revised the model—
incorporating an additional constuct called *cultural desire* and blended
in genetics, ethnopharmacology, and biocultural ecology in the construct of cultural knowledge. The resulting five interlocking circles
depicted the dynamism and interdependence among the five constructs. According to Campinha-Bacote (2002), all five constructs need
to be managed regardless of when the nurse comes into the interaction.
This second version's graphic representation could also be accesesed
on the Transcultural C.A.R.E. Web site.

Campinha-Bacote (2005a, 2007, 2008) further refined the construct
of cultural desire and represented the model of the process of cultural
competence as that of an erupting volcano. As such, Campinha-Bacote
(2011) highlighted the key role of cultural desire in the process of
becoming culturally competent. The third version's graphic representation could also be found on the Transcultural C.A.R.E. Web site. On
this graphic representation, cultural desire is at the base of a volcano.
Cultural awareness, encounters, knowledge, and skill are depicted as
the smoke emitted while the volcano smolders (Campinha-Bacote,
2003a, 2005a, 2007, 2008, 2011). In 2010, Campinha-Bacote started to
collect evidence-based research studies with her model and discovered

that cultural encounters is a "pivotal and key construct" (2011, para 4) in one's journey to cultural competence. The fourth graphic representation of *The Process of Cultural Competence in the Delivery of Healthcare Services* centered on cultural encounter; this also is available on Dr. Campinha-Bacote's Web site.

Campinha-Bacote (2003a, 2007, 2011) emphasized that cultural competence is a process of *becoming* and not a state of *being.* The values of caring and love for one another is the motivational factor for cultural competence. Recognizing that a component was missing in her model, Campinha-Bacote (2005a) pursued and completed a degree in theological studies; she thereafter included a biblical worldview in her Biblically Based Model of Cultural Competence.

In her model, Campinha-Bacote (2005a) stressed the call for personal sacrifice on our part—our biases and prejudices toward clients whose culture is other than our own—in order to foster cultural desire in ourselves. She acknowledged the difficulty of this sacrifice when we care for clients whose values, beliefs, and practices are in conflict with our own. In addition, Campinha-Bacote (2005a) advocated for the virtues of being teachable and of being humble: the former calls for attentiveness and willingness to learn from clients; the latter requires a lifelong value of self-evaluation as one partners with individuals, groups, and communities.

The self is vital as a starting point in the journey to cultural competence. Campinha-Bacote (2005a) defined cultural awareness "as the deliberate self-examination and in-depth exploration of one's own cultural background" (p. 27). Furthermore, this awareness requires intense self-assessment of one's biases, prejudices, and stereotypes directed to clients whose culture is different; this is aimed at preventing cultural imposition (Campinha-Bacote, 2005a).

According to Campinha-Bacote (2005a) and Purnell (2008), there are four levels of cultural competence: unconcious incompetence, concious incompetence, conscious competence, and unconcious competence. Health care providers have unconscious incompetence when they are unaware of lacking cultural knowledge while those who are conciously incompetent have the awareness of lacking that knowledge (Campinha-Bacote, 2005a). Consciously competent individuals have the knowledge and skill to provide culturally competent interventions; those who are unconciously competent have the automatic ability to render culturally competent care (Campinha-Bacote, 2005a).

The serious question of racism in health care must be acknowledged by health care professionals (Campinha-Bacote, 2002, 2003a,

2005a, 2007, 2011). Including self-awareness is the first step to prevention of discrimination and racism as a health care provider embarks on a journey to self-competence. Campinha-Bacote (2003a, 2007, 2011) further stressed that such personal journey is a process of becoming, not a state of being.

Assessing Levels of Cultural Competence

In order to provide culturally competent care, Campinha-Bacote (2007) suggests asking oneself whether the health care provider asked the right questions. Dr. Campinha-Bacote (2003a, 2007) developed the awareness, skill, knowledge, encounters, desire (ASKED) model where "A" stands for awareness, "S" for skill, "K" for knowledge, "E" for encounters, and "D" for desire.

In her Biblically based model of cultural competence, Dr. Campinha-Bacote (2005a) revised the question to *being asked* for one's readiness as a health care worker to appropriately care for a client. The "B" represents the bible; Campinha-Bacote (2005a) emphasized care from a biblical, Christian worldview, supporting the position of teaching "intellectual and moral virtues" (p. 19) and integrating these in her model.

In examining one's *awareness,* Campinha-Bacote reminds the nurse of personal biases and possible tendency for racism. In terms of *skill,* the question that the nurse must ask is the ability to conduct a cultural assessment (Campinha-Bacote, 2005a). In the area of *knowledge,* the question that needs to be asked refers to knowing different cultures and worldviews among people. Of *encounters,* Campinha-Bacote (2005a) refers to the numbers of face-to-face interactions with people from cultures different than one's own. Regarding *desire,* the resounding question to ask is whether or not one truly wants to become culturally competent (Campinha-Bacote, 2005a).

While the ASKED model is subjective, Campinha-Bacote (2010) suggests the use of the *Inventory for Assessing the Process of Cultural Competence Among Healthcare Professionals*—Revised (IAPCC-R) for formal self-assessment of level of cultural competence. She developed the IAPCC-Student Version (IAPCC-SV) to assess the cultural competence of student nurses. For her Biblical model, Campinha-Bacote (2005a) generated the *Inventory for Assessing Biblical Worldview of Cultural Competence Among Healthcare Professionals (IABWCC).* Both tools are available by contacting Dr. Campinha-Bacote at the C.A.R.E. Web site (http://www.transculturalcare.net).

The advent of quantifiable tools to measure the level of cultural competence is commendable. Administering such tools prior to and after implementation of educational programs could provide directions for implementation and could lead to better outcomes. These outcomes, along with government mandates and guidelines for prevention of disparities in health care—as well as standards from accrediting bodies for academic and practice institutions—could pave the way for more standardized integration of culturally competent care across settings in education, practice, and administration.

SECTION 2. APPLICATION OF THE MODEL IN NURSING EDUCATION

Although there has been agreement that the cultural competency component of nursing curricular content must include knowledge, skills, and attitudes, there are inconsistencies in terms of content, standards, and evaluation of outcomes (Campinha-Bacote, 2006, 2008; Lipson & Desantis, 2007). Furthermore, affective construct such as cultural desire has gotten little or no attention (Campinha-Bacote, 2003b, 2008). While clarifying ways of teaching cultural desire, Campinha-Bacote (2008) emphasized that this affective characteristic not only can be "caught" from peers, faculty, or workshop speakers but also could be taught in the curricula. In teaching cultural desire, Campinha-Bacote (2008) reminded us to address caring, love, sacrifice, humility, and compassion.

Wittig (2004) used Campinha-Bacote's (2003a) model to survey 28 associate senior degree nursing students regarding the knowledge, skills, and attitudes considered essential when providing culturally competent care for Native Americans. The findings indicated four areas of knowledge: general cultural factors; spiritual and religious beliefs; health and risk factors; and self-knowledge (Wittig, 2004). According to Wittig, two primary skill areas emerged from the study: basic nursing skills congruent with the Native American culture and effective communication skills. Furthermore, her participants identified two essential attitudes: (1) open-mindedness, being nonjudgmental, and caring; and (2) respect. This and similar surveys will provide directions to curricular development as more and more schools abide by the American Association of Colleges of Nursing (AACN, 1998, 1999, 2008) and National League of Nursing (NLN, 2009) mandates in preparing culturally competent graduates.

Kardong-Edgreen and Campinha-Bacote (2008) evaluated the use of the *Inventory for Assessing the Process of Cultural Competency Among Healthcare Professionals*—Revised (IAPCC-R) (Campinha-Bacote, 2007) among 212 students prior to graduation at four diverse U.S. baccalaureate nursing programs. The transcultural preparation of the students were diverse: two of the programs employ Leininger's theory and Campinha-Bacote's model; one program has a two-credit culture course; another integrates cultural content. The findings revealed that all 212 students scored only in the cultural awareness level; raising more questions such as reliability of the IAPCC-R and timing of evaluation at graduation versus later in practice (Kardon-Edgreen & Campinha-Bacote, 2008). Recently, Campinha-Bacote (2008) developed the IAPCC-SV to measure cultural desire among students; she recommends use of qualitative means such as journaling and field notes along with this quantitative tool. A replication of this study will give more insight to the development of cultural competence among nursing students. Table 3.1 illustrates the use of Campinha-Bacote's five constructs in a sample assignment of a

TABLE 3.1 A Sample Assignment of a Course in the Master's Program That Applies Campinha-Bacote's Model as Well as Current Research About Filipino Americans. May Be Adapted to Undergraduate or Doctoral Program

NUR 504-Transcultural Nursing	Credits: 3	Prerequisites: Nursing Research

Cultural awareness
  Am I aware of my personal biases against Filipino Americans?
  Are there research showing racist practices against this group?

Cultural knowledge
  Read
    de la Cruz, F., McBride, M., Compas, L. B., Calixto, P., & VanDerveer, C. P. (2002). White paper on the health status of Filipino Americans and recommendations for research. *Nursing Outlook, 50*(7), 7–15.

    Bjork, J. P., Cuthbertson, W., Thurman, J. W., & Lee, Y. S. (2001). Ethnicity, coping, and distress among Korean Americans, Filipino Americans, and Caucasian Americans. *Journal of Social Psychology, 14*(4), 421–442.

    Berg, J. (1999). The perimenopausal transition of Filipino American midlife women: Biopsychosociocultural dimensions. *Nursing Research, 48*(2), 71–77.

    Other relevant research

Cultural encounter
  Caring for Filipino Americans in practice settings
  Interview: First generation Filipino American
  • According to this book, Filipino Americans place high emphasis on_____. Is this correct according to your experiences and knowledge? If yes, please explain. If no, please add more information.
  • According to this article, Filipino Americans prefer to_____. Is this correct? If yes, please explain. If no, kindly add more information.

(Continued)

TABLE 3.1 *Continued*

NUR 504-Transcultural Nursing   Credits: 3   Prerequisites: Nursing Research

Cultural encounter
- According to the book(s) I reviewed, _____ are hesitant to sign organ donation cards. Is this true? If yes, please explain. If no, kindly add more information.
- Be creative in using variations of these questions.
- If you had asked some creative questions during the interviews, please include them.
- You may include the whole interview as an appendix at the end of the paper after the Reference list. Do include enough information on the *Brief Interview* portion of the paper.

Cultural skill
- Discuss a minimum of two research studies involving this group. Compare and contrast the research studies. Discuss strengths and limitations. Despite the weaknesses and limitations, are these research studies helpful in your case study and in your development of culturally competent care plan?
- Discuss culturally competent nursing interventions using Campinha-Bacote's Biblical model of cultural competence and findings from research studies.

Cultural desire
Do I want to be competent in caring for Filipino American clients. What is the next step in my journey? How do I sustain my desire to learn knowledge, skills, and competencies in caring for Filipino Americans and for other cultural groups?

nursing course at the master's level. This assignment could be used as a guide for any cultural group.

SECTION 3. APPLICATION OF THE MODEL IN NURSING PRACTICE

Campinha-Bacote's (2005a, 2005b, 2007, 2008) two models, *A Biblically based model of cultural competence* (2005a) and *The Process of Cultural Competence in the Delivery of Healthcare Services* (2007), could easily be applied to various practice settings. Many states require continuing education (CE) credits for renewal of registration. Annual self-learning via intranet or the internet or face-to-face modules are some of the common delivery methods for cultural competency training. Workshops by transcultural experts such as those of Campinha-Bacote (2010) are implemented by some hospitals and institutions to promote cultural competence among the staff. Other hospitals invite transcultural experts from nearby areas for workshops either as part of compliance with The Joint Commission's (TJC, 2010) *Advancing Effective Communication, Cultural Competence, and Patient and Family-Centered Care: A Roadmap for Hospitals* or as part of endeavors toward Magnet status (P. Sagar, personal communication, December 5, 2009; April 2010). There is some available research on cultural competence among health professionals using *The Process of Cultural Competence in the Delivery of Healthcare Services* (Campinha-Bacote, 2007).

In 2008, Capell, Dean, and Veestra examined the correlation between cultural competence and ethnocentrism among 27 physical therapists, 18 occupational therapists, and 26 nurses. Conducted in British Columbia, Capell and colleagues used Campinha-Bacote's IAPCC-R and the Generalized Ethnocentric Scale (GENE) by Neuliep (2002 as cited in Capell et al., 2008). Results indicated the following: (1) no significant difference in the IAPCC-R and the GENE across professional groups and (2) moderately strong correlation between cultural competence and ethnocentrism (Capell et al., 2008).

When designing CE bearing workshops, Campinha-Bacote's models of Cultural Competence may be used along with evidence-based and best practices among populations served by a specific hospital. Table 3.2 shows a sample workshop assignment in a 3-CE credits-approved course at Visionary Hospital, Anytown, USA, that applies Campinha-Bacote's model as well as current research about Korean Americans.

TABLE 3.2 A Sample Workshop Assignment in a 3-Continuing Education Credits–Approved Course at Visionary Hospital, Anytown, USA, That Applies Campinha-Bacote's Biblically Based Model of Cultural Competence as Well as Current Research About Korean Americans

Module 1: My Journey To Cultural Competence	Credits: 3 CE

Cultural awareness
Am I aware of my personal biases against Korean Americans?
Are there research showing racist practices against this group?

Cultural knowledge
Read
Bjork, J. P., Cuthbertson, W., Thurman, J. W., & Lee, Y. S. (2001). Ethnicity, coping, and distress among Korean Americans, Filipino Americans, and Caucasian Americans. *Journal of Social Psychology, 14*(4), 421–442.

Lee, E. E., & Farran, C. J. (2004). Depression among Korean, Korean Americans, and Caucasian American family caregivers. *Journal of Transcultural Nursing, 15*(1), 18–25.

Other relevant research articles

Cultural encounter
Patient care assignment of Korean Americans or
Interview: First generation Korean American
- According to this book, Korean Americans place high emphasis on_____. Is this correct according to your experiences and knowledge? If yes, please explain. If no, please add more information.
- According to this article, Korean Americans prefer to_____. Is this correct? If yes, please explain. If no, kindly add more information.
- According to the book(s) I reviewed, _____ are hesitant to sign organ donation cards. Is this true? If yes, please explain. If no, kindly add more information.

(Continued)

TABLE 3.2 *Continued*

Module 1: My Journey To Cultural Competence	**Credits: 3 CE**

Cultural encounter
- Be creative in using variations of these questions.
- If you had asked some creative questions during the interviews, please include them.
- You may include the whole interview as an appendix at the end of the paper after the Reference list. Do include enough on the *Brief Interview* portion of the paper.

Cultural skill
- Discuss a minimum of two research studies involving this group. Compare and contrast the research studies. Discuss strengths and limitations. Despite the weaknesses and limitations, are these research studies helpful in your case study and in your development of culturally competent care plan?
- Discuss culturally competent nursing interventions using Campinha-Bacote's Biblical model of cultural competence and findings from research studies.

Cultural desire
   Do I want to be competent in caring for Korean American clients? What is the next step in my journey? How do I sustain my cultural desire here and for other cultural groups?

SECTION 4. APPLICATION OF THE MODEL IN NURSING ADMINISTRATION

Nurse administrators are in key positions to promote cultural competence initiatives among health care workers. In academia, deans and chairs of nursing programs need to take the leadership to maximize the creation of separate courses in the undergraduate as well as graduate programs. If this is not possible due to a packed curriculum, the integration of cultural competence in all nursing and related courses needs to be guided by available toolkits (AACN, 2008; Galanti & Woods, 2007; NLN, 2009; TJC, 2010).

How Are We Doing?

On the ocassion of the 20th year anniversary since the American Nurses Association (1986) promulgated its initial guidelines on cultural diversity in nursing curricula, Dr. Campinha-Bacote (2006) posed this question: "... How are we doing 20 years later?" (p. 243). Five years later, the same question could be asked. In this 25-year journey of small steps, maybe we are further away in the process of ensuring that cultural diversity and cultural competence content, skills, and competencies are in our curricula; maybe we are not. Some nurse authors have developed tools to assess cultural competence among nurses but we lack valid and reliable tools to evaluate curricular outcomes (Campinha-Bacote, 2006). Tools for individual assessment of cultural competence such as the IAPCC-R, IABWCC, and the IAPCC-SV (Campinha-Bacote, 2003a, 2005a, 2007, 2011) could provide valid assessments as proven by research in academia and practice settings. Those assessments would be quite helpful in planning curricular approaches in both arenas.

On the other hand, the continuing international migration to the United States continues to generate interest in studying the relationship between acculturation and the health and health beliefs of immigrants (de la Cruz, Padilla, & Agustin, 2000). In spite of being the largest Asian group in California, the health status, treatment, and health care needs of Filipino Americans have not been generated (de la Cruz, McBride, Compas, Calixto, & VanDerveer, 2002). From *A Short Acculturation Scale for Hispanics*, de la Cruz et al. (2000) adapted and modified *A Short Acculturation Scale for Filipino Americans* (ASASFA). The ASASFA underwent forward translation; pretesting and committee review; back translation; pretesting and committee review; final expert review; and instrument validation yielding a mean acculturation score of 0.85 and an overall cronbach α coefficient for internal consistency at 0.85 (de la Cruz et al., 2000). The ASASFA may be used for planning recruitment, engagement, and retention of foreign educated Filipino nurses and other health professionals or for assessment in planning community partnerships and collaborations. It is also interesting to note the potential for adaptation and modification of the ASASFA for other ethnic groups.

Nurse administrators in the practice arena are faced with the same questions as nurse administrators in academia. It is imperative that organizational competence be assessed along with individual cultural competence. Tools with validity and reliability are now available such as the COA360 to measure organizational cultural competence (LaVeist, Relosa, & Sawaya, 2008).

Despite the fact that Transcultural Nursing society has offered international certification in TCN since 1988 (DeSantis & Lipson, 2007; Leininger & McFarland, 2002), there only are about 85 certified transcultural nurses to date (P. Sagar, personal communication, March 10, 2011; TCNS, 2011). Certification in TCN—in the United States and abroad—has not received recognition that is on par with other certifications, both in academia and administration (P. Sagar, personal communication, July 15, 2006). This may change in light of the intensifying focus on diversity, cultural competence, and attempts to narrow the gap in disparities among minorities in accessing and receiving quality of care. Nurse administrators in academia and practice are in strategic places to initiate, persist, and evaluate certification in TCN, both in the basic and advanced categories, respectively, among the nursing faculty and hospital nursing staff. When rewards and recognition are in place, nurses will have more incentives other than self-motivation and responsibility for their own continuing educational needs.

Case Study

Mercedes Lopez, Chief Nursing Officer at Bluesky Hospital is reviewing the proposed CE 2-hour lesson plan from the Director of Continuing Education (Appendix B). The CE calls for a budget for the continuing education of all levels of nurses at the hospital.

REFERENCES

American Association of Colleges of Nursing. (1998). *The essentials of baccalaureate education for professional nursing practice.* Washington, DC: Author.

American Association of Colleges of Nursing. (1999). *Nursing education's agenda for the 21st century.* Washington, DC: Author.

American Association of Colleges of Nursing. (2008). *Cultural competency in baccalaureate nursing education.* Washington, DC: Author.

American Nurses Association (1986). *Cultural diversity in nursing.* Kansas City, MO: ANA House of Delegates.

American Nurses Association. (1991). *Position statement on cultural diversity.* Kansas City, MO: Author.

Andrews, M. M., & Boyle, J. S. (2008). *Transcultural concepts in nursing care* (5th ed.). Philadelphia, PA: Wolters Kluwer/Lippincott Williams & Wilkins.

Berg, J. (1999). The perimenopausal transition of Filipino American midlife women: biopsychosociocultural dimensions. *Nursing Research, 48*(2), 71–77.

Bjork, J. P., Cuthbertson, W., Thurman, J. W., & Lee, Y. S. (2001). Ethnicity, coping, and distress among Korean Americans, Filipino Americans, and Caucasian Americans. *Journal of Social Psychology, 14*(4), 421–442.

Campinha-Bacote, J. (2002). The process cultural competence in the delivery of healthcare services: A model of care. *Journal of Transcultural Nursing, 13*(3), 181–184.

Campinha-Bacote, J. (2003a). *The process cultural competence in the delivery of healthcare services: A culturally competent model of care.* Cincinnati, OH: Transcultural C.A.R.E. Associates.

Campinha-Bacote, J. (2003b). Many faces: Addressing diversity in health care. *Journal of Issues in Nursing, 8*(1), 16–22. Retrieved November 16, 2010, from http://www.nursingworld.org/MainMenuCategories/ANAMarketplace/ANAPeriodicals/OJIN/TableofContents/Volume82003/No1Jan2003/AdressingDiversityinHealthCare.aspx

Campinha-Bacote, J. (2005a). *A Biblically based model of cultural competence in the delivery of healthcare services.* Cincinnati, OH: Transcultural C.A.R.E. Associates.

Campinha-Bacote, J. (2005b). A Biblically based model of cultural competence in healthcare delivery. *Journal of Multicultural Nursing & Health, 11*(2), 16–22.

Campinha-Bacote, J. (2006). How are we doing 20 years later? *Journal of Nursing Education, 45*(7), 243–244.

Campinha-Bacote, J. (2007). *The process of cultural competence in the delivery of healthcare services: The journey continues.* Cincinnati, OH: Transcultural C.A.R.E. Associates.

Campinha-Bacote, J. (2008). Cultural desire: "Caught" or "taught"? *Contemporary Nurse, 28,* 141–148.

Campinha-Bacote, J. (2010). *Transcultural training institute: Transcultural C.A.R.E. Associates.* Retrieved January 23, 2011, from http://transculturalcare.net/

Campinha-Bacote, J. (2011). *The process of cultural competence in the delivery of healthcare services.* Retrieved March 10, 2011, from http://transculturalcare.net/

Capell, J., Dean, E., & Veestra, G. (2008). The relationship between cultural competence and ethnocentrism of health care professionals. *Journal of Transcultural Nursing, 19*(2), 121–125.

de la cruz, F. A., Padilla, G. V., & Agustin, E. O. (2000). Adapting a measure of acculturation for cross cultural research. *Journal of Transcultural Nursing, 11*(3), 191–198.

de la Cruz, F., McBride, M., Compas, L. B., Calixto, P., & VanDerveer, C. P. (2002). White paper on the health status of Filipino Americans and resommendations for research. *Nursing Outlook, 50*(7), 7–15.

Desantis, L. A., & Lipson, J. G. (2007). Brief history of inclusion of content on culture in nursing education. *Journal of Transcultural Nursing, 18*(1), 7S–9S.

Galanti, G., & Woods, M. (2007). *Cultural sensitivity: A pocket guide for health care professionals.* Oakbrook Terrace, IL: Joint Commisssion Resources.

Giger, J. N., & Davidhizar, R. E. (2008). *Transcultural nursing: Assessment and intervention* (5th ed.). St. Louis, MO: Mosby Elsevier.

Kardong-Edgreen, S., & Campinha-Bacote, J. (2008). Cultural competency of graduating U.S. Bachelor of Science nursing students. *Contemporary Nurse, 28,* 37–44.

LaVeist, T. A., Relosa, R., & Sawaya, N. (2008). The COA360: A tool for assessing the cultural competency of healthcare organizations. *Journal of Healthcare Management, 53*(4), 257–266.

Lee, E. E., & Farran, C. J. (2004). Depression among Koren, Korean Americans, and Caucasian American family caregivers. *Journal of Transcultural Nursing, 15*(1), 18–25.

Leininger, M. M. (2002b). Culture care assessments for congruent competency practice. In M. Leininger & M. McFarland (Eds.), *Transcultural nursing: Concepts, theories, research, and practice* (3rd ed., pp. 117–143). New York, NY: McGraw-Hill Companies.

Leininger, M. M. (2006). Culture Care Diversity and Universality and evolution of the ethnonursing method. In M. Leininger and M. McFarland, *Culture care diversity and universality: A Worldwide nursing theory* (pp. 1–41). Sudbury, MA: Jones & Bartlett.

Leininger, M. M., & McFarland, M. R. (2002). Transcultural nursing: Curricular concepts, principles and teaching and learning activities for the 21st century. In M. Leininger & M. McFarland (Eds.), *Transcultural nursing: Concepts, theories, research, and practice* (3rd ed., pp. 527–561). New York, NY: McGraw-Hill Companies.

Leuning, C. J., Swiggum, P. D., Wiegert, H. M. B., & McCollough-Zander, K. (2002). Proposed standards for transcultural nursing. *Journal of Transcultural Nursing, 13*(1), 40–46.

Lipson, J. G., & Desantis, L. A. (2007). Current approaches to integrating elements of cultural competence in nursing education. *Journal of Transcultural Nursing, 18*(1), 10S–20S.

National League of Nursing. (2009). *A commitment to diversity in nursing and nursing education.* Retrieved January 26, 2011, from http://www.nln.org/aboutnln/reflection_dialogue/refl_dial_3.htm

Purnell, L. D. (2008). The Purnell model for cultural competence. In L. D. Purnel & B. J. Paulanka. *Transcultural health care: A culturally competent approach* (3rd ed., 19–55). Philadelphia, PA: FA Davis.

Spector, R. E. (2009). *Cultural diversity in health and illness* (7th ed.). Upper Saddle River, NJ: Pearson Education.

The Joint Commission. (2010). *Advancing effective communication, cultural competence, and patient and famuly-centered care: A roadmap for hospitals.* Oakbrook Terrace, IL: Author.

Transcultural Nursing Society. (2011). Transcultural nursing certification. Retrieved June 24, 2011, from http://www.tcns.org/Certification.html

Wittig, D. (2004). Knowledge, skills, and attitudes of nursing students regarding culturally congruent care of Native Americans. *Journal of Transcultural Nursing, 15* (1), 54–61.

NCLEX-TYPE TEST QUESTIONS (1–15)

1. When Leuning, Swiggum, Wiegert, and McCollough-Zander (2002) developed the standards for transcultural nursing, they used one of the following theoretical frameworks from a theory and model of:
   A. Leininger and Campinha-Bacote
   B. Purnell and Giger & Davidhizar
   C. Leininger and Andrews & Boyle
   D. Spector and Campinha-Bacote

2. Which of the following constructs did Campinha-Bacote include in 2005 to further refine her model?
   A. cultural awareness
   B. cultural knowledge
   C. cultural skill
   D. cultural desire

3. A team of researchers plans to use Campinha-Bacote's *Inventory for Assessing the Process of Cultural Competence Among Healthcare Professionals*—Student Version (IAPCC-SV). Which of the following statements by the team will best capture the breadth of cultural desire that may not be captured by quantitative tools alone?
   A. "We will also use the scoring system of the IAPCC-SV."
   B. "We will also use the T-test in addition to the scoring system of the IAPCC-SV."
   C. "We will also use the χ^2 in addition to the scoring system of the IAPCC-SV."
   D. "We will also use journaling and field notes in addition to the scoring system of the IAPCC-SV."

4. Both Campinha-Bacote and Purnell described four levels of cultural competence. Which one of the following does not belong to the four levels of cultural competence:
   A. unconciously incompetent
   B. conciously incompetent
   C. unconciously competent
   D. unconciously aware of incompetence

5. The nurse educator plans to use Campinha-Bacote's model in preparing the annually required cultural competence module for nurses. The nurse educator had administered Campinha-Bacote's *Inventory for Assessing a Biblical Worldview of Cultural Competence Among Healthcare Professionsals*. Of the 100 nurses in the hospital, 10 scored culturally competent. Which one of the following approaches will be more likely to honor cultural desire among the nurses?
   A. making the module available on the Intranet; to be completed by all 100 nurses
   B. making the module available on the Intranet; to be completed by 90 nurses, optional for 10 nurses
   C. making the module available on the Intranet; to be completed optionally by 100 nurses
   D. making the module available on the Intranet; to be completed after a pretest

6. In her graphic representation of the Biblical model of cultural competence, Campinha-Bacote designated cultural desire on which part of the erupting volcano?
   A. smoke
   B. lava
   C. base
   D. top

7. You are applying Campinha-Bacote's Biblical model of cultural competence in an assignment for an undergraduate nursing class. Which of the following statements best describes the construct of cultural desire?
   A. motivation of the nurse to engage in the process of cultural competence
   B. ability of the nurse to engage in the process of cultural competence
   C. skill of the nurse to engage in the process of cultural competence
   D. awareness of the nurse to engage in the process of cultural competence

8. You are applying Campinha-Bacote's Biblical model of cultural competence for a case study assignment in your doctoral nursing class. Which of the following statements best describes the construct of cultural awareness?
   A. cultural awareness is the self-examination of one's own cultural background
   B. motivation of the nurse to engage in the process of cultural competence
   C. ability of the nurse to engage in the process of cultural competence
   D. skill of the nurse to engage in the process of cultural competence

9. In Campinha-Bacote's *The Process of Cultural Competence in the Delivery of Healthcare Services*, she had coined the Awareness, Skill, Knowledge, Encounters, Desire (ASKED) mnemonic. According to Campinha-Bacote, which one of the following best describes the ASKED mnemonic?
   A. objective
   B. subjective
   C. both objective and subjective
   D. none of the above

10. When using Campinha-Bacote *The Process of Cultural Competence in the Delivery of Healthcare Services Model,* health care professionals seeking a more formal form of cultural competence self-assessment could use the:
    A. *Inventory for Assessing Process of Cultural Competence among Healthcare Professionals*—Student Version
    B. *Inventory for Assessing Process of Cultural Competence among Healthcare Professionals*—Biblical Version
    C. *Inventory for Assessing Process of Cultural Competence among Healthcare Professionals*—Revised
    D. *Inventory for Assessing Process of Cultural Competence among Healthcare Professionals*—Biblical

11. According to Campinha-Bacote, which one of the following is the best question to ask when reflecting on one's cultural desire?
    A. Do I have prejudices and biases?
    B. Do I really want to be culturally competent?
    C. Do I have the knowledge of the client's worldview?
    D. Do I have the skill to perform a cultural assessment of this group?

12. According to Campinha-Bacote, which one of the following is the best question to ask when reflecting on one's cultural skill?
    A. Do I have prejudices and biases?
    B. Do I really want to be culturally competent?
    C. Do I have the knowledge of the client's worldview?
    D. Do I have the skill to perform a cultural assessment of this group?

13. According to Campinha-Bacote, which one of the following is the best question to ask when reflecting on one's cultural knowledge?
    A. Do I have prejudices and biases?
    B. Do I really want to be culturally competent?
    C. Do I have the knowledge of the client's worldview?
    D. Do I have the skill to perform a cultural assessment of this group?

14. According to Campinha-Bacote, which one of the following is the best question to ask when reflecting on one's cultural encounters?
    A. How do I deal with my prejudices and biases?
    B. Do I really want to be culturally competent?
    C. How many face-to-face encounters have I had with culturally diverse clients?
    D. Do I have the skill to perform a cultural assessment of this group?

15. According to Campinha-Bacote, the process of cultural competence is a journey. As a journey, which of the following statements is NOT true about cultural competence?
    A. cultural competence is dynamic, not static
    B. cultural competence is a process of becoming, not being
    C. cultural competence is cyclic, not linear
    D. cultural competence is dynamic, a destination

(Answers to these questions can be found on p. 144)

4

JOYCE NEWMAN GIGER AND RUTH DAVIDHIZAR'S TRANSCULTURAL ASSESSMENT MODEL

SECTION 1. REVIEW OF THE MODEL

Dr. Joyce Newman Giger and Dr. Ruth Davidhizar (2002a, 2004, 2008) began their *transcultural assessment model* (GDTAM) in 1988 when there were few cultural asessment tools available, and in response to students' need to provide care to culturally diverse patients. In creating the GDTAM, Giger and Davidhizar (2002a) based their model on the seminal work of Dr. Leininger; on the work of Dr. Spector; on Orque, Bloch, and Monroy; and on Hall. In 1995, Giger and Strickland (as cited in Giger & Davidhizar, 2002a) tested the utility of the model through a $750,000 Department of Defense grant to explore behavioral risk reduction for African American premenopausal women with elevated risk for coronary artery disease.

The Giger and Davidhizar (2008) model has five metaparadigms:

- "transcultural nursing and culturally diverse nursing;
- culturally competent care;
- culturally unique individuals;
- culturally sensitive environments;
- health and health status based on culturally specific illness and wellness behavior" (p. 5).

In the GDTAM, transcultural nursing (TCN) is defined as "a culturally competent practice field that is client centered and research focused" (Giger & Davidhizar, 2008, p. 5). Nurses must use TCN knowledge as a skill and an art to provide care to diverse populations in a culturally appropriate and competent manner, taking into consideration GDTAM's six cultural phenomena. The model views cultural competence as a dynamic process implemented by an individual or health care agency by using significant interventions based on the client's "cultural heritage, beliefs, attitudes, and behaviors" (Giger & Davidhizar, 2008, p. 6). Each individual has unique beliefs, cultural norms, and experiences; achieving cultural competence enables the nurse to develop meaningful interventions in promoting health among individuals (Giger & Davidhizar, 2002a, 2008). Culturally competent care can and should be rendered in diverse settings and in all levels of care: primary, secondary, and tertiary. The GDTAM is presented in Figure 4.1, illustrating the ability to give every individual a unique identity. Figure 4.2 expands each area of the six cultural phenomena and specifically tunes in on assessment focus and questions to ask clients across cultures.

Giger and Davidhizar (2004, 2008) had consistently presented the content of their textbook *Transcultural Nursing: Assessment and Interventions* throughout its five editions into two parts: (1) theory portion with an introduction followed by six chapters discussing each of the cultural phenomena, and (2) application of the six phenomena in the assessment and care of individuals from diverse cultures. According to Glittenberg (2002), this textbook has added to the evolution of TCN and to the field that it is today. Initially published in 1991, the textbook was translated to French and is adopted by schools in French-speaking countries (Davidhizar, Giger, & Hannenpluf, 2006). In 1998, Giger and Davidhizar published a companion book (Davidhizar & Giger, 1998; Davidhizar et al., 2006), *Canadian Transcultural Nursing: Assessment and Intervention* featuring cultural groups throughout Canada.

Six Cultural Phenomena

When using the GDTAM, six cultural phenomena are evaluated, namely, *biological variations, environmental control, time, social orientation, space,* and *communication* (Dowd, Davidhizar, & Giger, 1998; Giger & Davidhizar, 1998, 2002a, 2002b, 2004, 2008). Although occuring in all cultures, each phenomenon is related to each other; overlaps with one another; and varies in its application and uses (Dowd, Davidhizar, et al., 1998). In addition, GDTAM offers a thorough assessment tool vital in the planning of care consistent with the individual needs of clients (American Association of Colleges of Nursing [AACN], 2008).

Physical characteristics such as stature and skin and hair color; enzymatic and genetic presence of diseases; susceptibility to illness; and

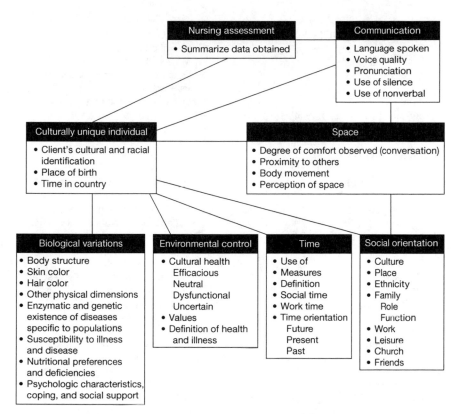

FIGURE 4.1 Giger and Davidhizar Transcultural Assessment Model.
Source: Reprinted from Giger, J. N., & Davidhizar, R. E. (2008). *Transcultural nursing: Assessment and intervention* (5th ed.). St. Louis, MO: Mosby Elsevier. Copyright Elsevier Mosby.

psychological coping comprise the areas for assessment of *biological variations* (Giger & Davidhizar, 2004, 2008). Many studies concerning growth and development and nutrition were conducted among White participants; hence prevailing norms are not reflective of racial variations.

When evaluating *environmental control*, Giger and Davidhizar (2004, 2008) include health care practices, values, and views on health and illness, including how one's behavior affected one's health. People with internal locus of control believe that the power to affect change is within; those with external locus of control believe in fate and luck (Giger & Davidhizar, 2008).

With the phenomenon of *time*, the assessment parameters are the nature of time and its measures; social time; work time; and time orientation whether past, present, or future. Cultures that identify with the past honor tradition and are respectful of elders. Present time orientation is characterized by living in the present; future orientation tends

CULTURALLY UNIQUE INDIVIDUAL
1. Place of birth
2. Cultural definition
   What is...
3. Race
   What is...
4. Length of time in country (if appropriate)

COMMUNICATION
1. Voice quality
   A. Strong, resonant
   B. Soft
   C. Average
   D. Shrill
2. Pronunciation and enunciation
   A. Clear
   B. Slurred
   C. Dialect (geographical)
3. Use of silence
   A. Infrequent
   B. Often
   C. Length
      (1) Brief
      (2) Moderate
      (3) Long
      (4) Not observed
4. Use of nonverbal
   A. Hand movement
   B. Eye movement
   C. Entire body movement
   D. Kinesics (gestures, expression, or stances)
5. Touch
   A. Startles or withdraws when touched
   B. Accepts touch without difficulty
   C. Touches others without difficulty
6. Ask these and similar questions:
   A. How do you get your point across to others?
   B. Do you like communicating with friends, family, and acquaintances?
   C. When asked a question, do you usually respond (in words or body movement, or both)?
   D. If you have something important to discuss with your family, how would you approach them?

SPACE
1. Degree of comfort
   A. Moves when space invaded
   B. Does not move when space invaded
2. Distance in conversations
   A. 0 to 18 inches
   B. 18 inches to 3 feet
   C. 3 feet or more
3. Definition of space
   A. Describe degree of comfort with closeness when talking with or standing near others
   B. How to objects (e.g., furniture) in the environment affect your sense of space?
4. Ask these and similar questions:
   A. When you talk with family members, how close do you stand?
   B. When you communicate with coworkers and other acquaintances, how close do you stand?
   C. If a stranger touches you, how do you react or feel?
   D. If a loved one touches you, how do you react or feel?
   E. Are you comfortable with the distance between us now?

SOCIAL ORGANIZATIONS
1. Normal state of health
   A. Poor
   B. Fair
   C. Good
   D. Excellent
2. Marital status
3. Number of children
4. Parents living or deceased?
5. Ask these and similar questions:
   A. How do you define social activities?
   B. What are some activities you enjoy?
   C. What are your hobbies, or what do you do when you have free time?
   D. Do you believe in a Supreme Being?
   E. How do you worship that Supreme Being?

FIGURE 4.2 Giger and Davidhizar Transcultural Assessment Model: Applications Across Cultures. (Figure continues on the next 2 pages)
Source: Reprinted from Giger, J. N., & Davidhizar, R. E. (2008). *Transcultural nursing: Assessment and intervention.* (5th ed.). St. Louis, MO: Mosby Elsevier. Copyright Elsevier Mosby.

F. What is your function (what do you do) in your family unit/system?

G. What is your role in your family unit/system (father, mother, child, advisor)?

H. When you were a child, what or who influenced you most?

I. What is/was your relationship with your siblings and parents?

J. What does work mean to you?

K. Describe your past, present, and future jobs.

L. What are your political views?

M. How have your political views influenced your attitude toward health and illness?

TIME
1. Orientation to time
   A. Past-oriented
   B. Present-oriented
   C. Future-oriented
2. View of time
   A. Social time
   B. Clock-oriented
3. Physiochemical reaction to time
   A. Sleeps at least 8 hours a night
   B. Goes to sleep and wakes on a consistent schedule
   C. Understands the importance of taking medication and other treatments on schedule
4. Ask these and similar questions:
   A. What kind of timepiece do you wear daily?
   B. If you have an appointment at 2 pm, what time is acceptable to arrive?
   C. If a nurse tells you that you will receive a medication in "about a half hour," realistically, how much time will you allow before calling the nurses' station?

ENVIRONMENTAL CONTROL
1. Locus-of-control
   A. Internal locus-of-control (believes that the power to affect change lies within)
   B. External locus-of-control (believes that fate, luck, and chance have a great deal to do with how things turn out)
2. Value orientation
   A. Believes in supernatural forces
   B. Relies on magic, witchcraft, and prayer to affect change
   C. Does not believe in supernatural forces
   D. Does not rely on magic, witchcraft, or prayer to affect change
3. Ask these and similar questions:
   A. How often do you have visitors to your home?
   B. Is it acceptable to you for visitors to drop in unexpectedly?
   C. Name some ways your parents or other persons treated your illnesses when you were a child.
   D. Have you or someone else in your immediate surroundings ever used a home remedy that made you sick?
   E. What home remedies have you used that worked? Will you use them in the future?
   F. What is your definition of "good health"?
   G. What is your definition of illness or "poor health"?

BIOLOGICAL VARIATIONS
1. Conduct a complete physical assessment noting:
   A. Body structure (small, medium, or large frame)
   B. Skin color
   C. Unusual skin discolorations
   D. Hair color and distribution
   E. Other visible physical characteristics (e.g., keloids, chloasma)
   F. Weight
   G. Height
   H. Check lab work for variances in hemoglobin, hematocrit, and sickle cell phenomena if Black or Mediterranean

FIGURE 4.2 (*Continued*) Giger and Davidhizar Transcultural Assessment Model: Applications Across Cultures.

2. Ask these and similar questions:
   A. What diseases or illnesses are common in your family?
   B. Has anyone in your family been told that there is a possible genetic susceptibility for a particular disease?
   C. Describe your family's typical behavior when a family member is ill.
   D. How do you respond when you are angry?
   E. Who (or what) usually helps you to cope during a difficult time?
   F. What foods do you and your family like to eat?
   G. Have you ever had any unusual cravings for:
      (1) White or red clay dirt?
      (2) Laundry starch?
   H. When you were a child what types of foods did you eat?
   I. What foods are family favorites or are considered traditional?

NURSING ASSESSMENT
1. Note whether the client has become culturally assimilated or observes own cultural practices.
2. Incorporate data into plan of nursing care:
   A. Encourage the client to discuss cultural differences; people from diverse cultures who hold different world views can enlighten nurses.
   B. Make efforts to accept and understand methods of communication.
   C. Respect the individual's personal need for space.
   D. Respect the rights of clients to honor and worship the Supreme Being of their choice.

   E. Identify a clerical or spiritual person to contact.
   F. Determine whether spiritual practices have implications for health, life, and well-being (e.g., Jehovah's Witnesses may refuse blood and blood derivatives; an Orthodox Jew may eat only kosher food high in sodium and may not drink milk when meat is served).
   G. Identify hobbies, especially when devising interventions for a short or extended convalescence or for rehabilitation.
   H. Honor time and value orientations and differences in these areas. Allay anxiety and apprehension if adherence to time is necessary.
   I. Provide privacy according to personal need and health status of the client (NOTE: the perception of and reaction to pain may be culturally related).
   J. Note cultural health practices:
      (1) Identify and encourage efficacious practices.
      (2) Identify and discourage dysfunctional practices.
      (3) Identify and determine whether neutral practices will have a long-term ill effect.
   K. Note food preferences:
      (1) Make as many adjustments in diet as health status and long-term benefits will allow and that dietary department can provide.
      (2) Note dietary practices that may have serious implications for the client.

FIGURE 4.2 (*Continued*) Giger and Davidhizar Transcultural Assessment Model: Applications Across Cultures.

to place more emphasis in setting objectives and plans for the future. Time orientation has a significant implication; for example, preventive health care necessitates future orientation since it involves future rewards (Giger & Davidhizar, 2002a, 2004, 2008).

The area of *social orientation* calls for culture, race, ethnicity as well as family role and function, friendships, hobbies, and belonging in other social institution such as the church. When children grow and learn a particular culture, it is somewhat a prison; Giger and Davidhizar (2008) refer to this as "culture bound"(p. 68). When an illness is tied to this phenomenon, it is called "culture-bound illness" (Giger & Davidhizar, 2008, p. 69). On the whole, people tend to be ethnocentric, viewing one's own way as the best. Health care professionals need to be respectful of other's beliefs and ways of life.

Space evaluation includes the comfort observed when space is invaded, distance from others, and notion of space. Personal space includes both the physical area surrounding the person's body as well as the inner space, which includes the spirit core (Scott, 1988, as cited in Giger & Davidhizar, 2008). Territoriality "refers to feelings or attitudes towards one's personal area" (Giger & Davidhizar, 2002a, p. 185). Refusal of care may result when a client feels a violation of one's personal space. The space needs of individuals vary from culture to culture.

Giger and Davidhizar (2008) refer to communication as a " . . . continuous process by which one person may affect another through written or oral language, gestures, facial expressions, body language, space, or other symbols" (p. 20). Barriers in communication are intensified when the nurse and client are from different cultures.

Communication has received more attention with the increasing focus by *Healthy People 2010 and 2020* (U.S. Department of Health and Human Services [USDHHS], 2001, 2011), the publication of the *Culturally and Linguistically Appropriate Services* (CLAS) (USDHHS, Office of Minority Health [OMH], 2001), *Advancing Effective Communication, Cultural Competence, and Patient- and Family-Centered Care: A Roadmap for Hospitals,* and the Florida study on *Cultural and Linguistic Care in Area Hospitals* (The Joint Commission [TJC], 2010a,b). Widely accepted as vital in navigation of health care, language is a prime factor in health care access.

In 1993, Spector integrated the six cultural phenomenon in her *cultural heritage model*, creating a holistic framework for culturally competent care (Giger & Davidhizar, 2004, 2008; Spector, 2004, 2009). Also in 1993, the National League for Nursing (NLN) published *Nursing Management Skills: A Modular Self-Assessment Series, Module 4, Transcultural Nursing;* this outlined the application of the GDTAM in learning and refining mangerial skills (Giger & Davidhizar, 2004, 2008). The NLN (2005, 2009b) again used Giger–Davidhizar's GDTAM as a framework in its *Core Competencies of Nurse Educators With Task Statements* as well as its *Diversity Toolkit*. AACN (2008) used the GDTAM along with three other models and a nursing theory in the preparation of *Cultural Competency in Baccalaureate Nursing Education* end of program competencies and faculty toolkit.

SECTION 2. APPLICATION OF THE MODEL IN NURSING EDUCATION

More than ever, there are now specific guidelines and mandates regarding the integration of diversity and cultural competence in nursing curricula to fulfill accreditation requirements and the demand of an increasingly diverse practice arena: AACN (1998, 1999, 2008); NLN (2005, 2009a, 2009b); American Nurses Association (1991, 1995, 2003); and TJC (2010a,b), formely the Joint Commission on the Accreditation of Healthcare Organizations. Standards of the Commission on Collegiate Nursing Education and the NLN Accrediting Commission stipulate adherence to its parent organizations' essential documents for all nursing programs. While some test items on diversity and cultural competence are part of the National Council Licensure Examination (NCLEX), State Boards of Nursing have not thoroughly integrated questions addressing cultural diversity and cultural competence (Pacquaio, 2007).

The Giger–Davidhizar (2002a, 2004, 2008) GDTAM is practical and straightforward, lending itself very well to application in nursing academia (Davidhizar & Giger, 2001; Davidhizar, Giger, et al., 2006) and health-related fields such as medical imaging, dental hygiene, and others (Dowd, Giger, & Davidhizar, 1998; Ryan, Carlton, & Ali, 2000). The GDTAM is integrated in all nursing programs at Bethel College, Indiana (Davidhizar & Giger, 2001; Eshelman & Davidhizar, 2006), Ball State University, Indiana, and Cox College, Misouri, whereas Georgia State University uses the GDTAM in selected courses (Lipson & Desantis, 2007). At the University of Alabama in Birmingham, the GDTAM is used only in MS courses that are supported by a Health Resources Services Administration (HRSA) grant (Lipson & Desantis, 2007). *Transcultural Nursing: Assessment and Interventions*, first published in 1991 and currently in its fifth edition, has been used as a textbook and as a framework integrated in nursing programs as well as other health care fields (Davidhizar & Giger, 2001; Glittenberg, 2002). In addition, Davidhizar and Giger (2001) reiterated the need for the whole faculty to be involved in the selection of a TCN textbook if it will be used througout the curriculum as well as in the decision to adopt a model or pick eclectic components from models to use in different nursing courses.

Registered nurses (RNs) with associate and diploma degrees receive little education in caring for diverse patients and working with diverse health care workers (Eshelman & Davidhizar, 2006). For this reason, Eshelman and Davidhizar (2006) called attention to the formation of a programmatic outcome in RN to Bachelor of Science in Nursing programs in the area of cultural sensitivity and fostering of cultural competence. Furthermore, Eshelman and Davidhizar emphasized the use of well-planned teaching strategies that could be employed in RN-BS programs such as story telling, article critiques, cultural analysis, cultural dinners, guest speakers, and international health exercises. Stories—such as fairy tales, personal and fictitious stories, puppet, and role playing—could assist in enhancing student listening skills and data collection and development of critical thinking (Eshelman & Davidhizar, 2006). Story telling as a narrative pedagogy provides opportunities to explore concepts from diverse points of view; to promote reflection; and to enhance affective learning and caring (Billings & Halstead, 2005). Critiquing literature guided by a set of critieria from faculty could facilitate discussion of cultural issues amid current events, guidelines, regulation, and mandates. The cultural analysis strategy involves a guided interview of a person from another culture; students bring their analysis along with a culinary specialty of the interviewee to class for comparative discussions. Guest speakers from diverse cultures, immigrants, and missionaries are invited; this develops cultural awareness and sensitivity (Eshelman & Davidhizar, 2006). The international health exercise consists of a description of one international community in terms of strengths and resources, health problems, and cultural implications.

In 2007, Hughes and Hood described one baccalaureate nursing program in the midwest using the Giger–Davidhizar model across the curriculum. Subsequent measurement of student cross-cultural interaction with the Freeman's (1993, as cited in Hughes & Hood, 2007) Cross-Cultural Evaluation Tool (CCET) yielded consistent increase in scores in all levels of the curriculum. Since the CCET only measures attitudinal and behavioral changes (Hughes & Hood, 2007), a tool that measures knowledge, skills, and competence may yield a more comprehensive result. Using a TCN model and determining its outcome from across courses and levels of nursing may be the best way to measure changes in student knowledge, skills, and competencies. The progress may be slow but there is intensifying attention now—more than ever—in the role of cultural competence to reduce health disparities.

Role Playing: Its Role in Enhancing Cultural Competence

Shearer and Davidhizar (2003) illustrated the application of the GDTAM in role-playing activities to foster cultural competence among nursing students. Role playing has a long history in nursing education. In role play, individuals enter upon the role of someone else while observers analyze and interpret (Billings & Halstead, 2005) enabling suggestions of new behaviors prior to the actual interaction (Shearer & Davidhizar, 2003). The role of the faculty centers on identifying objectives for the experience; providing time frame and guidelines including various roles; monitoring the process; and facilitating analysis and debriefing (Billings & Halstead, 2005; Gaberson & Oermann, 1999; Shearer & Davidhizar, 2003). When debriefing after the role play, it is imperative that the educator include learning outcomes from the experience, application to practice, further learning needed, feelings generated, and changes needed to improve patient care (Gaberson & Oermann, 1999). Students' creativity is tapped in role-playing acitivities. The freedom to be creative and spontaneous favors the learning of new behavior; for this reason, role play is usually limited to 15 to 20 minutes and with brief roles to be portrayed (Billings & Halstead, 2005; Gaberson & Oermann, 1999). This behavior could be used not only with cognitive and psychomotor domains but also with affective objectives in teaching and learning.

Opportunities for students to comment facilitate critical thinking and exploration of the many possible interpretations of the situation (Shearer & Davidhizar, 2003). Furthermore, role playing may be used in all levels of programs from licensed practical to doctoral programs. The six essential areas in GDTAM could be applied in various role-playing scenarios, in its totality or by selecting specific areas. Furthermore, the GDTAM has been used as an assessment model to provide culturally competent care to peoples of different cultures. In the following role-playing scenarios, TCN knowledge about culturally competent care to Muslim patients will be applied (Giger & Davidhizar, 2002b; Wehbe-Alamah, 2006, 2008).

Sample Role Play Scenario

Student A: She was dressed as a Muslim woman with loose fitting clothes; she had temporarily removed her head covering while washing up. A basin with water was in front of her. She had a fresh change of clothes beside her on the bed. She was planning to pray in her room later and would be requesting the nurse to move her bed to face Mecca. Her prayer rug was on the floor. When she saw the nurse rushing into the room, she scrambled to place her head cover. She was anxious to know about the composition of the gelatin pills; some of them, she said, had pork ingredient and she is a devout Muslim who adheres to Muhammad's rule. Her face clouded over when the nurse stated that there is no way the bed could be moved to face east; the nurse said this without even an explanation.

Student B: She was dressed in blue scrubs as a nurse. The nurse went right into the room without knocking, carrying a medication tray with two gelatin pills. She offered the pills to the patient, adding that the doctor just ordered it during that morning's round. The nurse was unaware that gelatin has pork components and did not offer to look it up or consult the pharmacist. She, without apparent thought and reflection, stated that there is no chance of moving the client's bed to face east. She seemed in a rush and did not explain nor apologized for the inability to grant the patient's request.

Reflection

Student C: He was dressed in a laboratory coat and will act as the facilitator, moderating the discussion following the role play. Following are some guide questions as previously discussed with faculty:

1. How is communication as a cultural phenomenon involved here? Discuss.
2. How is biological variations as a cultural phenomenon involved here? Discuss.
3. How is space as a cultural phenomenon involved here? Discuss.
4. Reenact the scenario.

Instructor/Educator: Debriefing

1. Reflect on the role play. How did you feel?
2. Discuss what you learned. What other learning needs do you have? Discuss.
3. Discuss the clinical application of this role play.
4. Examine the changes needed in your own knowledge, skills, and behavior in order to incorporate culturally congruent care.

SECTION 3. APPLICATION OF THE MODEL IN
NURSING PRACTICE

The six essential areas—or any of the areas—of Giger and Davidhizar's (2002a, 2002b, 2004, 2008) GDTAM could be built around existing admission assessment tool in any client care setting or in planning care for culturally diverse individuals. The GDTAM is used all over the world and provides an assessment tool to obtain baseline data regarding a specific cultural group. While there is variation within cultures as much as across cultures, the baseline assessment is an "excellent starting point" in providing culturally competent care (Giger & Davidhizar, 2002b, p. 85). For example, in an existing tool, *communication* could be added, followed by "primary language spoken"; "primary language when reading"; or if an interpreter is needed, the "dialect spoken and most understood." When using an interpreter, assessing the primary dialect or language is vital prior to requesting for an interpreter onsite or accessing the language line. As an example, a Filipino American patient whose dialect is Bicol (mid-southern Philippines) may have more difficulty with Pilipino (national language in the Philippines) than with another client whose dialect is Tagalog (basis for Pilipino).

Ensuring that communication is included becomes a necessity when there is a marked increase in the U.S. population—from 31.8 million (1990) to 47 million (2000) (OMH, USDHHS, 2001)—among individuals who speak languages other than English at home. TJC (2010b) figure for these non-English speakers are 17.9% (2000) and 19.6% (2006–2008) of the U.S. population. CLAS standards 4 through 7 mandate language access services (LAS) for non-English speaking clients and for clients with limited English proficiency (LEP) in institutions receiving federal funding (OMH, USDHHS, 2001). Admittedly, language is a vital area when navigating the health care services (TJC, 2010a) and problems in this area could create further disparities in access and quality of care among minorities and diverse populations.

Case Scenario

The nurse educator has assigned a junior nursing student to care for a Pakistani client who has LEP. The nurse educator and student nurse are working with the client's primary nurse. Upon accessing the language line and specifying that the client is from Pakistan, the nurse educator was promptly connected to an Urdu interpreter. At the end of the session, the interpreter advised that, for future interpretation needs, the nurse must request for a Punjabi instead of an Urdu interpreter since the patient speaks more Punjabi than Urdu. In this case, being mindful of inquiring about languages and dialects spoken in certain countries or regions in a country would be helpful prior to using the language line or any medical interpreters.

Review the above scenario and *Cultural and Linguistic Care in Area Hospitals* (TJC, 2010b). After careful review of this document, answer the questions below.

Questions for Reflections

1. How well do you know the LAS at the clinical site?
2. Discuss the use of the LAS by various members of the health team such as the physician, nurse, social worker, and pharmacist. Who uses it most? Why?
3. Explain why effective communication is vital in navigating health care systems.

Every health care institution uses some method of care planning for clients. The GDTAM could be a framework in developing and integrating culturally competent care plans for diverse clients. While policy and procedure manuals abound in health care institutions, most of the procedures do not contain modifications for culturally diverse clients (P. L. Sagar, personal communication, February 2, 2011). As a ready reference, a copy of *Transcultural Nursing: Assessment and Intervention* (Giger & Davidhizar, 2008), along with other TCN books and pocket guides must be available on each unit as well as in the library. TJC's (2007, 2010a,b) guidelines, research, development of resources, and inclusion of cultural competence among its standards for accreditation will further pave the way for integration of diversity in health care policies and procedure guidelines among individual organizations.

One other area in which the GDTAM could be applied in practice settings is end-of-life care. As the United States gets more culturally diverse, it becomes imperative that health care professionals possess the knowledge and skills for rituals and other aspects of end-of-life care (Giger, Davidhizar, & Fordham, 2006). Some cultural groups have difficulty and reluctance in the area of advanced directives such as the Hispanics (Giger et al., 2006) and Filipino Americans (McAdams, Stotts, Padilla, & Puntillo, 2005, as cited in Vance, 2008). Illustrating how the GDTAM can be used in end-of-life care, Giger et al. (2006) called upon nurses to use cultural understanding, respect, and sensitivity when planning, implementing, and evaluating care for the dying patient and the family. Pain experience and expression vary among cultural groups; as such, the nurse needs to individualize assessment and plan of care. Some people see pain as punishment for wrongdoing in the past. While some cultures believe that people should not suffer, others believe that it is a test of faith and people must carry on (Giger et al., 2006). The nurse's understanding, creativity, and sensitivity are indeed vital when assisting clients and families and or significant others.

SECTION 4. APPLICATION OF THE MODEL IN NURSING ADMINISTRATION

The GDTAM may easily be used in learning and refining managerial skills (Dowd, Davidhizar, et al., 1999; Giger & Davidhizar, 2004, 2008), developing policies and procedure manuals, in orientation process of new nurses—including those from other countries. Currently, as hospitals and health care facilities downsize, many health care managers find themselves jobless. The six cultural phenomena provide a simple tool for managers in planning the potential fit of the new job location (Dowd, Davidhizar, et al., 1999). For example, in terms of environmental control, people with internal locus of control perceive themselves as authority whereas those with external locus of control view others as authority figures. Hence, managers who tend to be authoritarian could face some difficulty in a setting where the staff expect the administrator to be facilitative (Dowd, Davidhizar, et al., 1999).

Nurses From Overseas

Brunero, Smith, and Bates (2008) examined the needs and experiences of 150 overseas qualified nurses in Sydney, Australia, working at a tertiary hospital. Australia, like the United States, is experiencing nursing shortages predicted to be about 41,000 in 2010 and had resorted to hiring foreign nurses. Brunero et al. (2008) acknowledged the previous work of Davidhizar, Dowd, and Giger (1999) wherein the GDTAM was used as a framework to guide administrator's role in assisting a diverse workforce through the use of the six cultural phenomena. Results from the 150 surveyed (56 returned the questionaires) revealed three themes: career and lifestyle opportunities, differences in practice, and homesickness (Brunero et al., 2008), related to the cultural phenomena of communication, space, environmental control, and social organization. The use of the GDTAM could creatively assist in the hiring and retention of overseas nurses. Table 4.1 shows application of the GDTAM in planning an orientation program for new Filipino nurses.

Nursing Education Administration

In nursing education administration, the dean of the school is in key position to facilitate integration of diversity and promotion of cultural competence in all programs; ensuring that academic policies are appropriate for all students, including culturally diverse students; and hiring, engagement, and retention of culturally diverse faculty and staff. Specifically, entire faculty involvement when selecting a model to use across programs or in selection of a textboook or textbooks to use (Eshelmann & Davidhizar, 2006) is in the purvue of the dean in larger schools or chair of the program in smaller colleges.

The are unique challenges and needs among culturally diverse nursing students. The six cultural phenomena may be used as a guide in planning interventions for recruitment, engagement, and retention of diverse students such as assistance with English comprehension, bridging technique, and faculty/student mentoring (Davidhizar & Shearer, 2005). Assisting with comprehension of English may include simple course directions, facilitation with networking, provision of

TABLE 4.1 Application of the Giger and Davidhizar's GDTAM's Six Cultural Phenomena to Plan Orientation of New Nurses From the Philippines

Communication	Are questions asked spontaneously or after trust is fostered?
	Are concerns offered spontaneously or in response to questions?
Space	Describe comfortable distance from patients, other nurses, other individuals.
Time	What is the acceptable reporting for business time?
	What is the acceptable reporting for social time?
Environmental control	What is the nurse's belief in terms of health? Illness? Treatment? Recovery?
Social organization	How close is the nurse to other family members? How is the nurse coping with homesickness?
Biological variation	What is the health status of the nurse?
	When sick, what is the belief in terms of notification of supervisor or reporting to work?
	Does the nurse feel that illness should not preclude one from working?

Source: Developed from Giger, J. N., & Davidhizar, R. E. (2008). *Transcultural nursing: Assessment and intervention* (5th ed.). St. Louis, MO: Mosby Elsevier.

concrete learning aids, and help with medical terminology. In the bridge technique according to Yoder (as cited in Davidhizar & Shearer, 2005), students are encouraged to hold on to their ethnic identity while faculty modify culturally appropriate teaching and learning modalities. Faculty mentors assist in the bridging activities; student mentors, having been successful in the bridging process, are useful to the students (Davidhizar & Giger, 2005).

REFERENCES

American Nurses Association. (1991). Position statement on cultural diversity in nursing practice. Kansas City, MO: Author.

American Nurses Association. (1995). *Nursing's social policy statement.* Washington, DC: Author.

American Nurses Association. (2003). *Nursing's social policy statement* (2nd ed.). Washington, DC: Nurses Books.

American Association of Colleges of Nursing. (1998). *The essentials of baccalaureate education for professional nursing practice.* Washington, DC: Author.

American Association of Colleges of Nursing. (1999). *Nursing education's agenda for the 21st century.* Washington, DC: Author.

American Association of Colleges of Nursing. (2008). *Cultural competency in baccalaureate nursing education.* Washington, DC: Author.

Billings, D. M., & Halstead, J. A. (2005). *Teaching in nursing: A guide for faculty* (2nd ed.). St. Louis, MO: Elsevier Saunders.

Brunero, S., Smith, J., & Bates, E. (2008). Expectations and experiences of recently recruited overseas qualified nurses in Australia. *Contemporary Nurse, 28*(1), 101–110.

Davidhizar, R. E., Dowd, S. B., & Giger, J. N. (1999). Managing diversity in the health care workplace. *The Health Care Supervisor, 17,* 51–62.

Davidhizar, R. E., & Giger, J. N. (1998). (Eds.). *Canadian transcultural nursing: Assessment and intervention.* Louis, MO: Mosby.

Davidhizar, R. E., & Giger, J. N. (2001). Teaching culture within the nursing curriculum using the Giger–Davidhizar model of transcultural nursing assessment. *Journal of Nursing Education, 40*(6), 282–284.

Davidhizar, R. E., Giger, J. N., & Hannenpluf, L. W. (2006). Your continuing education topic 3 2005: Using the Giger–Davidhizar transcultural assessment model (GDTAM) in providing patient care. *The Journal of Practical Nursing, 56*(1), 20–26.

Davidhizar, R. E., & Shearer, R. (2005). When your nursing student is culturally diverse. *Health Care Manager, 240*(4), 356–363.

Dowd, S. B., Giger, J. N., & Davidhizar, R. E. (1998). Use of Giger and Davidhizar's transcultural assessment model by health professions. *International Nursing Review, 45*(4), 119–122, 128.

Dowd, S. B., Davidhizar, R. E., & Giger, J. N. (1998). Will you fit if you move to a job in another culture? *Health Care Manager, 18*(2), 20–27.

Eshelman, J., & Davidhizar R. E. (2006). Strategies for developing cultural competency in an RN-BS program. *Journal of Tanscultural Nursing, 17*(2), 179–183.

Gaberson, K. B., & Oermann, M. H. (1999). *Clinical teaching strategies in nursing.* New York, NY: Springer.

Giger, J. N., & Davidhizar, R. E. (2002a). The Giger and Davidhizar transcultural assessment model. *Journal of Transcultural Nursing, 13*(3), 185–188.

Giger, J. N., & Davidhizar, R. E. (2002b). Culturally competent care: Emphasis on understanding the people of Afghanistan, Afghanistan Americans, and Islamic culture and religion. *International Council of Nurses, International Nursing Review, 49,* 79–86.

Giger, J. N., & Davidhizar, R. E. (2004). *Transcultural nursing: Assessment and intervention* (4th ed.). St. Louis, MO: Mosby Elsevier.

Giger, J. N., & Davidhizar, R. E. (2008). *Transcultural nursing: Assessment and intervention* (5th ed.). St. Louis, MO: Mosby Elsevier.

Giger, J. N., & Davidhizar, R. E., & Fordham, P. (2006). Multi-cultural and multi-ethnic considerations and advanced directives: Developing cultural competency. *Journal of Cultural Diversity, 13*(1), 3–9.

Hughes, K. H., & Hood, L. J. (2007). Teaching methods and an outcome tool for measuring cultural sensitivity in undergraduate nursing students. *Journal of Transcultural Nursing, 18*(1), 57–62.

Lipson, J. G., & Desantis, L. A. (2007). Current approaches to integrating elements of cultural competence in nursing education. *Journal of Transcultural Nursing, 18*(1), 10S–20S.

Shearer, R. G., & Davidhizar, R. (2003). Using role play to develop cultural competence. *Journal of Nursing Education, 42*(6), 273–276.

National League for Nursing. (2005). *Core competencies of nurse educators with task statements.* New York, NY: Author. Retrieved January 26, 2011, from NLN website: http://www.nln.org/aboutnln/core_competencies/cce_dial3.htm

National League for Nursing. (2009a). *A commitment to diversity in nursing and nursing education.* Retrieved January 26, 2011, from NLN website: http://www.nln.org/aboutnln/reflection_dialogue/rfl_dial3.htm

National League for Nursing. (2009b). *Diversity toolkit.* Retrieved January 26, 2011, from NLN website: http://www.nln.org/aboutnln/reflection_dialogue/rfl_dial3.htm

Pacquaio, D. (2007). The relationship between cultural competence education and increasing diversity in nursing schools and practice settings. *Journal of Transcultural Nursing, 18*(1), 28S–370S.

The Joint Commission. (2010a). *Advancing effective communication, cultural competence, and patient- and family-centered care: A roadmap for hospitals.* Oakbrook Terrace, IL: Author.

The Joint Commission. (2010b). *Cultural and linguistic care in area hospitals.* Oakbrook Terrace, IL: Author

U.S. Department of Health and Human Services, Office of Minority Health. (2000). *Culturally and linguistically appropriate services.* Retrieved August 26, 2010, from http://www.usdhhs.gov

U.S. Department of Health and Human Services. *Healthy People 2020*. Retrieved 12 January, 2011, from http://www.healthypeople.gov/HP2020/Objectives/selectionCriteria.aspx

Vance, A. R. (2008). Filipino Americans. In J. N. Giger & R. E. Davidhizar (Eds.), *Transcultural nursing: Assessment and intervention* (5th ed., pp. 467–493). St. Louis, MO: Mosby Elsevier.

Wehbe-Alamah, H. M. (2006). Generic care of Lebanese Muslim women in the Midwestern USA. In M. M. Leininger and M. R. McFarland (Eds.), *Culture care diversity and universality: A worldwide nursing theory* (pp. 307–325). Sudbury, MA: Jones & Bartlett.

Wehbe-Alamah, H. (2008). Bridging generic and professional care practices for Muslim patients through use of Leininger's culture care modes. *Contemporary Nurse, 28*(1), 83–97.

NCLEX-TYPE TEST QUESTIONS (1–15)

1. When applying the Giger and Davidhizar transcultural assessment model (GDTAM), the nurse asks her Navajo client: "Could you describe what you usually do when your blood sugar is high?" Which of the following areas of the GDTAM is the nurse assessing?
   A. communication
   B. time
   C. social orientation
   D. environmental control

2. The nurse is caring for a Mexican American client who has diabetic gangrene of one of his toes. The nurse asks the client: "Please describe to me how decision is made in your family." The area of Giger and Davidhizar's GDTAM being assessed is:
   A. communication
   B. time
   C. social orientation
   D. environmental control

3. Which of the following statements would be most therapeutic when assessing the need for an interpreter while admitting a Filipino American client who has limited English proficiency?
   A. "Tell me what dialect you use when speaking and reading."
   B. Do tell me what dialect you use when speaking and reading."
   C. Please tell me what dialect you use when speaking and reading."
   D. "What dialect do you use when speaking and reading?"

4. The Vietnamese client states: "In my home, the family has an altar honoring our ancestors." The most likely time orientation of this client is:
   A. past
   B. present
   C. future
   D. both present and future

5. The new pediatric nurse remarked to the nurse manager: "The Hmong child that I just admitted looks very small for his age." Which of the following comments by the nurse manager best explains biological variations?
   A. "Most growth charts are normed among Caucasian children."
   B. "Let us make a referral to Child Protective Services."
   C. "Most growth charts are normed among non-Asian children."
   D. "Let us make a referral to the nutritionist for evaluation."

6. The client stated that the baby is sick because someone had cast the "evil eye" on her. This is an example of Giger and Davidhizar's assessment area of:
   A. social orientation
   B. environmental control
   C. biological variations
   D. communication

7. The nurse is caring for a 13-year-old African American child with sickle cell crisis. Which of the following planned interventions show the nurse's knowledge of the pain this client is experiencing?
   A. Administer pain medication as needed only. Promptly assess for pain relief.
   B. Administer pain medication round the clock. Promptly assess for pain relief.
   C. Administer pain medication as needed only. Promptly assess for pain relief every hour.
   D. Administer pain medication as needed only. Promptly assess for pain relief every 4 hours.

8. When integrating Giger and Davidhizar's area of social orientation in the hospital admission tool, the transcultural nurse will include which of the following areas?
   A. notion of space; distance when interacting with others; family roles and functions
   B. health care practices; views on health and illness; belonging in social institutions
   C. notion of time; family roles and functions; belonging in social institutions
   D. race, ethnicity; family roles and functions; belonging in social institutions

9. While conducting an orientation for newly arrived nurses from China, the nurse educator at a medical center noted that the nurses were avoiding eye contact. Avoidance of eye contact may be an expression of:
   A. social orientation
   B. invasion of space
   C. respect for authority
   D. discomfort

10. The nurse noticed that her client from Great Britain pulls away and steps back as they were talking in the hallway. Based on the Giger and Davidhizar's transcultural assessment model, the area that the nurse is performing is:
    A. time
    B. space
    C. communication
    D. social organizations

11. The transcultural nurse is implementing role playing in her continuing education session for a group of health care workers. Which of the following statements best describe the advantage of role playing as a teaching and learning modality?
    A. suggestion and exploration of new behavior after the actual interaction
    B. suggestion and exploration of new behavior before the actual interaction
    C. suggestion and exploration of new behavior simultaneous with the actual interaction
    D. suggestion and exploration of prior behavior before the actual interaction

12. The nurse administrator is collaborating with the transcultural nurse in planning retention strategies for new nurses from Mexico. The nurse administrator had contracted with the community college nearby to offer English as a Second Language (ESL) course onsite at the hospital. Which statement by the nurse administrator will be more therapeutic when presenting this idea to the Mexican nurses?
    A. The ESL classes will begin tomorrow; the classes will assist in your speaking and writing abilities.
    B. The ESL classes will assist in your speaking and writing abilities; do write five reasons how it would enhance your nursing practice.
    C. The ESL classes will assist in your speaking and writing abilities; please write five reasons how it would enhance your nursing practice.
    D. The ESL classes are mandatory; the classes will assist in your speaking and writing abilities.

13. The nurse is teaching her diabetic Mexican American client self-administration of insulin. The nurse noticed that the patient kept forgetting to cleanse the site with alcohol pad. Which of the following statements by the nurse is the most therapeutic?
    A. "You are doing it wrong. Let me show you the corect way."
    B. "Cleansing the site is important to prevent infection. Let me show you the corect way."
    C. "You are doing it wrong. Let me show you the corect way."
    D. "Cleansing the site is important to prevent infection. You are doing it wrong."

14. The clinic nurse noticed that the Chilean American client is 30 minutes late for his appointment. When asked, he replied that a friend of his who he had not seen in months had dropped by and he forgot about the time. Giger and Davidhizar explain this as a time orientation that is:
    A. future
    B. present
    C. past
    D. both present and past

15. While discharging a Puerto Rican client, the nurse discusses medication regimen at home. Which of the following will the client most likely remember about a medication that needs to be taken three times a day?
A. "Take the medication with your breakfast, lunch, and dinner."
B. "Take the medication every 6 hours during the day."
C. "Take the medication in the morning, afternoon, and evening."
D. "Take the medication every 4 hours during the day."

(*Answers to these questions can be found on p. 145*)

5

RACHEL SPECTOR'S HEALTH TRADITIONS MODEL

SECTION 1. REVIEW OF THE MODEL

Spector's (2004a, 2009) *health traditions model* (HTM) integrates Ester and Zitzow's theory on how an individual's lifestyle mirrors his/her own traditional culture. Spector views heritage consistency on a continuum indicating "consistent heritage (traditional) and an inconsitent heritage (acculturated)" (2004a, p. 8). Spector used three aspects of heritage consistency: culture, ethnicity, and religion in 2004 and added acculturation and socialization in 2008 as she refined her model. Individuals with more traditional heritage are more observant of traditions; those who are more acculturated show less observance (American Association of Colleges of Nursing [AACN], 2008; Spector, 2002, 2004a, 2009). The HTM was officially created in 1994; the Immigrant Health Traditions exhibit was mounted in that year at Ellis Island Immigration Museum, Jersey City, New Jersey (Spector, 2002). Serving as a gateway for countless immigrants to the United States, Ellis Island and the Statue of Liberty are symbols of beacons of opportunity that comes when migrating to this country. While Ellis Island's (2010) function as gateway was officially ended in 1954, its exhibits bring nostalgia, compassion, and connectedness for immigrants in general. Being at Ellis Island is a strong reminder of the roots for many succeeding generations when reflecting about family pioneers who braved the seas (or the air and land) to come and settle on this land that "is paved in gold." It is right and fitting that a nursing transcultural model be among the Ellis Island exhibit. When integrating transcultural nursing (TCN) concepts in nursing curricula, a trip to see Lady Liberty and the exhibits at Ellis Island could be an assignment for reflection.

In discussing cultural competence, Spector (2004a, 2009) emphasizes its interconnectedness with culture and with demographics, immigration, and poverty. In order to safely deliver *Culture Care*, health care professionals have to undergo a complex process to develop knowledge, skills, and attitude (Spector, 2009). Consequently, Spector (2009) poses these thought-provoking questions:

- "How do you *really* inspire people to hear the content;
- How do you liberate providers from the burdens of prejudice, xenophobia...racism, ethnocentrism...?" (p. xii)

Spector (2004a, 2009) arranged the content of *Cultural Diversity in Health and Illness* into four parts: foundations of cultural competency; health, illness, and heritage; selected populations' beliefs and practices and health care issues; and an epilogue applying the knowledge in health care delivery, planning, and education for both health professionals and patients. The four parts of her textbook is set amid globalization, current mandates and guidelines, and other developments in the panorama of health care. Originally published in 1977 as a promise to her nursing students, Spector's (2002, 2004a, 2009) textbook had undergone seven editions.

Spector (2004a, 2009) compares culture to a luggage that each individual carries along throughout his/her life and passes on to the next generation. Each luggage is filled with learned values, beliefs—all the tangibles and intangibles—that individuals learned through socialization. According to Spector (2009), ethnicity indicates the following characteristics that groups share: "geographic origin, migratory status, race, language and dialect, religion, traditions, food preferences ... " (p. 12). In relation to ethnicity, Spector (2009) cited ethnocentrism as the notion of superiority pertaining to one's ethnic group and xenophobia as the "morbid fear of strangers" (p. 12). Foreign-born persons may have increased ethnic affiliation while in the process of acculturation or in the journey of self-acceptance. Religion, as a component of heritage, is the faith in the divine power that governs the universe (Spector, 2004a, 2009). Following religious teachings, for many people, promotes spirituality and health. In many cultures, illness is viewed as punishment for nonadherence to religious codes. The concepts in Spector's (2002) model are interconnected, signifying the difficulty of traditional people and immigrants when accessing health care delivery.

Health Traditions Model

In 1993, Spector (2004a, 2004b, 2009) incorporated Giger and Davidhizar's six cultural phenomena of environmental control, biological variations, social organization, communication, space, and time orientation to form the *health traditions model* (Davidhizar & Giger, 1998; Giger & Davidhizar, 2004a, 2008). This unique model (Figure 5.1) provides a holistic framework for assessment and provision of culturally competent care and first appeared in Potter and Perry's *Fundamentals of Nursing* textbook (Davidhizar & Giger, 1998; Giger & Davidhizar, 2008). Spector (2004a, 2009) refers to this model as *personal health traditions of a unique cultural being* (PHTUCB).

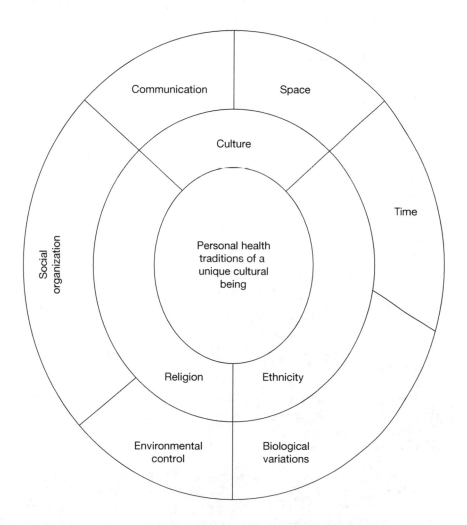

FIGURE 5.1 Spector's Personal Health Traditions of a Unique Cultural Being.
Source: Reprinted with permission from Spector, R. E. (2009). *Cultural Diversity in Health and Illness* (7th ed.). Upper Saddle River, NJ: Pearson Prentice Hall. Copyright Pearson Education.

In addition, Spector (2004b) coined the term *culture care,* "a concept that describes professional health care that is culturally sensitive, culturally appropriate, and culturally competent" (p. v). To determine the depth of identification with one's own personal heritage, Spector also developed a *heritage assessment tool* (Figure 5.2).

Heritage Assessment Tool

This set of questions can be used to investigate a given patient's or your own ethnic, cultural, and religious heritage. It can help you to perform a heritage assessment to determine how deeply a given person identifies with a particular *tradition*. It is most useful in setting the stage for understanding a person's HEALTH traditions. The greater the number of positive responses, the greater the person's identification with a traditional heritage. The one exception to positive answers is the question about family name change. This question may be answered negatively.

1. Where was your mother born? _____
2. Where was your father born? _____
3. Where were your grandparents born?
   (1) Your mother's mother? _____
   (2) Your mother's father? _____
   (3) Your father's mother? _____
   (4) Your father's father? _____
4. How many brothers _____ and sisters _____ do you have?
5. What setting did you grow up in? Urban _____ Rural _____ Suburban _____
6. What country did your parents grow up in?
   Father _____
   Mother _____
7. How old were you when you came to the United States? _____
8. How old were your parents when they came to the United States? Mother _____ Father _____
9. When you were growing up, who lived with you? _____
10. Have you maintained contact with
    a. Aunts, uncles, cousins? (1) Yes _____ (2) No _____
    b. Brothers and sisters? (1) Yes _____ (2) No _____
    c. Parents? (1) Yes _____ (2) No _____
    d. Your own children? (1) Yes _____ (2) No _____
11. Did most of your aunts, uncles, cousins live near your home?
    (1) Yes _____ (2) No _____
12. Approximately how often did you visit your family members who lived outside your home?
    (1) Daily _____ (2) Weekly _____ (3) Monthly _____ (4) Once a year or less _____
    (5) Never _____

FIGURE 5.2 Spector's Heritage Assessment Tool (*Continued*).

Source: Reprinted with permission from Spector, R. E. (2004b). *Cultural care guide to heritage assessment and health traditions* (3rd ed.). Upper Saddle River, NJ: Pearson Prentice Hall. Copyright Pearson Education.

13. Was your original family name changed?
    (1) Yes _____ (2) No _____

14. What is your religious preference?
    (1) Catholic _____ (2) Jewish _____ (3) Protestant _____ (4) Denomination _____
    (5) Other _____ (6) None _____

15. Is your spouse the same religion as you?
    (1) Yes _____ (2) No _____

16. Is your spouse the same ethnic background as you?
    (1) Yes _____ (2) No _____

17. What kind of school did you go to?
    (1) Public _____ (2) Private _____ (3) Parochial _____

18. As an adult, do you live in a neighborhood where the neighbors are the same religion and ethnic background as yourself?
    (1) Yes _____ (2) No _____

19. Do you belong to a religious institution?
    (1) Yes _____ (2) No _____

20. Would you describe yourself as an active member?
    (1) Yes _____ (2) No _____

21. How often do you attend your religious institution?
    (1) More than once a week _____ (2) Weekly _____ (3) Monthly _____
    (4) Special holidays only _____ (5) Never _____

22. Do you practice your religion at home?
    (1) Yes _____ (2) No _____ (If yes, please specify) (3) Praying _____
    (4) Bible reading _____ (5) Diet _____ (6) Celebrating religious holidays _____

23. Do you prepare foods of your ethnic background?
    (1) Yes _____ (2) No _____

24. Do you participate in ethnic activities?
    (1) Yes _____ (2) No _____ (If yes, please verify) (3) Singing _____
    (4) Holiday celebrations _____ (5) Dancing _____ (6) Festivals _____
    (7) Costumes _____ (8) Other _____

25. Are your friends from the same religious background as you?
    (1) Yes _____ (2) No _____

26. Are your friends from the same ethnic background as you?
    (1) Yes _____ (2) No _____

27. What is your native language? _____

28. Do you speak this language?
    (1) Prefer _____ (2) Occasionally _____ (3) Rarely _____

29. Do you read your native language?
    (1) Yes _____ (2) No _____

FIGURE 5.2 (*Continued*). Spector's Heritage Assessment Tool.

Spector (2004b), who sometimes refers to the HTM as health traditions assessment model, views health as "the state of balance within the body, mind, and spirit, and with the family, community, and the forces of the natural world (p. 17)." The body, mind, and spirit each have three dimensional aspects with three facets each, resulting in nine interrelated aspects of health: maintenance, protection, and restoration (Spector, 2002). This holistic approach may see more utility in health care as complementary alternative methods such as acupuncture, yoga, and meditation not only gain more use but also reveal, through research, their quantifiable benefits in promoting wellness and in the treatment and rehabilitation of some illnesses.

The AACN (2008) used the HTM with three other models and a nursing theory in the preparation of *cultural competency in baccalaureate nursing education* end-of-program competencies and faculty toolkit. Spector's book has been used by nursing schools as an organizing framework when they prefer not to use a specific model (Lipson & Desantis, 2007) and has been credited for "adding to the evolution of transcultural nursing" (Glittenberg, 2004, p. 7).

SECTION 2. APPLICATION OF THE MODEL IN NURSING EDUCATION

As discussed in the previous chapter, Spector incorporated Giger and Davidhizar's transcultural assessment model (GDTAM) into the HTM in 1993; this unique model provides holistic framework for assessment and provision of culturally competent care. Spector had created a table that could serve as quick reference when caring for diverse clients (Davidhizar & Giger, 1998; Giger & Davidhizar, 2004, 2008). According to Spector (2004a, 2009), the PHTUCB is a depiction of how cultural phenomena affect an individual with unique ethnic, religious, and cultural background. Such focus on uniqueness of each individual is an ever-present reminder to health professionals to avoid stereotyping when dealing with culturally diverse clients.

In undergraduate programs in nursing, students obtain the basic requisite knowledge and skills in foundation courses. The use of the PHTUCB can be a useful framework as beginning nursing students journey into acquiring knowledge, skills, and competencies in caring for diverse populations and interacting with diverse health care workers. When integrating transcultural concepts in the curriculum, we must be mindful of the complex healing systems of our clients and communities (Spector, 2004a, 2009). These healing systems are vital if we were to act as bridge between this healing sytem and the professional system. Further use of the framework in progressive nursing courses could provide consistency as students acquire and gain more proficiency in applying TCN principles while caring for diverse clients and collaborating with diverse health care workers. Spector's *Cultural Care Guide to Heritage Assessment and Health Traditions* (2004b) could be a portable pocket guide for students and practitioners.

Spector (2002) had emphasized the advocacy role of the nurse in terms of patient's health maintenance, protection, and restoration. This advocacy role could be threaded into all courses and all the levels of the nursing curriculum, in itself or with the six concepts of the GDTAM. Table 5.1 illustrates how this could be used in community health nursing when planning health education for a Mexican migrant workers' community.

TABLE 5.1 Application of Spector's Model in Planning Health Education for a Migrant Community

	Physical	**Mental**	**Spiritual**
Health maintenance	Where and how do you access health care providers?	What do you do for recreation? Do you have games, books, magazines, or television programs that are culture specific?	Are there resources to meet your spiritual needs? How far are churches from the migrant community?
Health protection	Do you have special clothes worn for protection? Where can you obtain them?	What activities do you need to avoid? Are there places that you need to avoid?	Where do you get special amulets? What for and when do you wear those? Do you have special spiritual practices?
Health restoration	Who are the traditional healers in the community? If they are not available in the immediate communty, where do you go? Do you use any traditional remedies? Where do you buy them? Are you able to grow herbs or other remedies?	Are there special teas, other drinks, or food that you use? Where would you obtain them?	Do you use folk healers? Are they available in the community?

Source: Developed from Spector, R. E. (2004b). *Cultural care guide to Heritage Assessment and Health Traditions* (3rd ed.). Upper Saddle River, NJ: Pearson Prentice Hall.

TABLE 5.2 Addendum to Existing or New Assessment Tool Incorporating Spector's Personal Health Traditions of a Unique Cultural Being

Cultural group	Were you born in the United States? ____if not, how old were you when you came to the United States?
Religion	Do you belong to a religious institution? Where do you usually pray? Would you prefer to see the clergy during hospitalization? Do you have any dietary limitations because of religion?
Communication	What is your native language? Do you speak and read English? ____ How long have you spoken English?
Nutrition	What is your preferred diet? Do you have any food allergy? Do you prepare ethnic foods? ____ Would you need special utensils in food preparation? ____

SECTION 3. APPLICATION OF THE MODEL IN NURSING PRACTICE

There is agreement that the United States is getting more diverse. Yet many assessment tools in clinical settings have few items related to cultural assessment. While there is much focus in medical assessment, there is little that pertains to the mind and spirit. Since the PHTUCB (Spector, 2004a, 2009) is holistic, its six cultural phenomena (Giger & Davidhizar, 2002a, 2004, 2008), along with the client's culture, religion, and ethnicity, as areas in totality or selectively, may be integrated into the existing assessment tools or used as reference in developing new assessment tools (Table 5.2). Government mandates and accreditation standards for cultural competence call for tools that would be effective in assessment, planning, implementation, and evaluation of care for culturally diverse patients.

SECTION 4. APPLICATION OF THE MODEL IN NURSING ADMINISTRATION

Spector's model could be applied to promote individual and organizational cultural competence. In the section about health care delivery and issues, Spector (2009) effectively outlined two points: (1) the health care provider's culture and (2) issues in health care delivery. Both factors immensely affect access to health care and, eventually, health disparities in the United States.

Health care providers such as nurses, physicians, dietitians, physical and occupational therapists, and other health team members are generally xenophobic and ethnocentric when it comes to beliefs regarding health and illness (Spector, 2009). The health care system has its own culture with its own language that would be strange and not understandable by the general public; words such as "nothing by mouth (NPO), shortness of breath (SOB), keep vein open (KVO), as soon as possible (ASAP), against medical advice (AMA)" are usually parts of health care workers' vocabulary. This contributes to some people's perception that the health care system is alien. In addition, Spector (2009) quoted the underlying norm that "all must be done to save a patient" regardless of wishes or financial catastrophe on the part of the family" (p. 169) and resulting in escalating health care costs.

In illustrating her point, Spector (2009) traced the issue of the per capita escalating cost of health care in selected years from 1960 to 2004 in the United States compared to other developed countries such as Norway, Spain, and Portugal. The United States has the highest cost at $6,102; in contrast, Norway ($3,966), Spain ($2,094), and Portugal ($1,824) have much lower costs (National Health Statistics [NHS] in 2007 as cited in Spector, 2009, pp. 172–174). In addition, Spector (2009) pointed out that while the cost is monumental, the outcomes do not justify the expenditures; for instance, the number of infant deaths in 2004 and the corresponding ranking compared to the same countries are as follows: The United States (6.8; 29th), Norway (3.2; 5th), Spain (3.5; 7th), and Portugal (4; 10th). The United States lags behind Cuba, which has 5.8 infant deaths in 2004 and ranked 27th among other countries (Spector, 2009).

During cyclical nursing shortages, U.S. hospitals have resorted to recruitment of foreign nurses. According to the National Sample Survey of Registered Nurses, of the total 3,063,163 of nurses in the United States, an estimated 170,235 completed their initial nursing degree in another country (United States Department of Health and Human Services [USDHHS], 2010). Close to half of these foreign educated nurses are from the Philippines (48.7%) while the rest are from the following countries: Canada (11.5%), India (9.3%), the United Kingdom (5.8), Korea (2.6%), Nigeria (2.0%), and other (17.3%) (USDHHS, 2010). In its position statement regarding the ethical recruitment of nurses, the International Council of Nurses (ICN) in 2007 acknowledged the right of registered nurses to migrate and seek better working conditions and opportunities. However, the ICN (2007) denounces the nurse drain that leaves inadequate health care in the nurses' coutry of origin. Foreign nurses, however, are entitled to appropriate orientation, supervision, and mentoring (ICN, 2007). Studies about the experiences, professional adjustment, acculturation, and retention rates of these foreign nurses need to be done. The following case study applies Spector's HTM in the orientation of new nurses from India.

Case Study

Visionary Hospital (VH), Anytown, USA, is in the process of hiring 35 new nurses from India. The Chief Nurse Officer (CNO) of VH traveled to Mumbai and personally interviewed and selected the nurses; the nurses will arrive in a month. All 35 nurses took the National Council Licensure Examination (NCLEX) in Mumbai and had passed. Out of the 35 nurses, 25 scored more than 500 in the Test for English as a Second Language (TOEFL) whereas the remaining 10 obtained scores between 400 and 475. English as a Second Language classes are contracted with the community college nearby; classes will be given onsite at the VH. Although the nurses scored high in TOEFL, it is anticipated that slang, colloquialism, and other factors would be areas of concern. The National Association of Indian Nurses of America (NAINA), in a city 300 miles, has been contacted by the CNO of the hospital. The NAINA president and other officers plan to come to the hospital and welcome the nurses. The NAINA is planning a one-on-one mentoring for the new nurses although their membership numbers present a problem. The AIANA only has 20 members. Belonging to the National Coalition of Ethnic Minority Nurses Association (NACEMNA), they had enlisted the help of the other associations under the coalition. The Philippine Nurses Association of America (PNAA) regional chapter already offered to help in the mentoring process. The NAINA plans to accept the PNAA's offer of assistance in the mentoring process, believing that although there is much difference between Asian Indian and Filipino American cultures, there are similarities in the experience of foreign nurses when they immigrate to a new country and work as professional nurses. Furthermore, both groups did not have mentoring when they arrived 10 to 25 years ago. Individually, these nurses recall the intense homesickness, painful process of acculturation, and difficulty with English language despite having been able to speak the language back home as part of their educational process.

Each nurse was surveyed with this Form A in Mumbai during the time of contract signing and the processing of immigration period. The Director of Nursing Education (DNE) is collating the findings and will be using these to plan how to meet the needs of the nurses as well as other retention activities for the new nurses. The DNE and her staff are using the best evidence available regarding alleviation of the nursing shortage, acculturation of foreign nurses, retention strategies, and promotion of cultural competence among health care workers. Table 5.3 illustrates the use of the model in the orientation of the new nurses from India.

TABLE 5.3 The Use of the Model in the Orientation of the New Nurses

Name: _____   Survey Form : A

Directions: Please take time to answer this survey. Your thoughtfulness and thoroughness will assist us in planning to make resources available for you as you make your adjustment as professional nurses in the United States. Many thanks for your time.

	Physical	Mental	Spiritual
Communication	What is your native language? How long have you spoken English? TOEFL Score _____	How comfortable are you in speaking English? Very comfortable _____ Comfortable _____ With some discomfort _____	What language or dialect do you use to pray?
Social organizations	Do you participate in ethnic activities? Yes ___ No ___ Specify: Singing _____ Dancing _____ Other _____	Do you anticipate homesickness? When you start feeling homesick how would you alleviate it?	Do you have any family in this area? Friends? In any part of the United States? Do you know any of the other nurses that you came with from India?
Health maintenance	Do you have preferences in terms of health care providers? Where and how would you access health care? Are there any dietary limitation(s)? Explain.	What do you do for recreation? Do you have games, books, tapes, magazines, or television programs that are culture specific?	Are there resources that you need to meet your spiritual needs? Explain. Do you belong to any temple or church? Are there any special holidays that you need to observe?
Health protection	Do you have special clothes worn for protection? Where can you obtain them?	What activities do you need to avoid? Are there places that you need to visit? Places that you need to avoid?	Where do you get special amulets? What for and when do you wear those? Do you have special spiritual practices?
Health restoration	Who are the traditional healers in the community? If they are not available in the immediate community, where would you go? Do you use any traditional remedies? Where do you buy them? Are you able to grow herbs or other remedies?	Are there special teas, other drinks, or food that you use? Where would you obtain them? Are there any dietary limitation(s)?	Do you use folk healers? If they are not available in the community face-to-face, is there a way to contact them by phone or online?

Source: Adapted from Spector, R. E. (2004b). Cultural care guide to heritage assessment and health traditions (3rd ed.). Upper Saddle River, NJ: Pearson Prentice Hall.

Another plan is to offer continuing education (CE) credits for nurses regarding Anglo Americans. More than 95% of the population within 300 miles of the hospital are Anglo Americans, with the remaining 5% distributed: about 2% American Indians, 2% Asian Indians, and 1% African Americans. The chief executive officer of the hospital works closely with the DNE and the chief medical officer as they plan succeeding CE offerings to help in the acculturation process of the nurses as well as to continue on the initiative to educate all health care workers.

REFERENCES

American Association of Colleges of Nursing. (2008). *Cultural competency in baccalaureate nursing education.* Washington, DC: Author.

Davidhizar, R. E., & Giger, J. N. (1998). *Canadian transcultural nursing: Assessment and intervention.* St. Louis, MO: Mosby.

Giger, J. N., & Davidhizar, R. E. (2002a). The Giger and Davidhizar transcultural assessment model. *Journal of Transcultural Nursing, 13*(3), 185–188.

Giger, J. N., & Davidhizar, R. E. (2008). *Transcultural nursing: Assessment and intervention* (5th ed.). St. Louis, MO: Mosby Elsevier.

Glittenberg, J. (2004). A transdisciplinary, transcultural model for health care. *Journal of Transcultural Nursing, 15*(1), 6–10.

International Council of Nurses. (2007). *Ethical nurse recruitment position paper.* Retrieved September 17, 2009, from http://www.icn.ch/psrecruit01.htm#_ftn1

Lipson, J. G., & Desantis, L. A. (2007). Current approaches to integrating elements of cultural competence in nursing education. *Journal of Transcultural Nursing, 18*(1), 10S–20S.

Spector, R. E. (2002). Cultural diversity in health and illness. *Journal of Transcultural Nursing, 13*(3), 197–199.

Spector, R. E. (2004a). *Cultural diversity in health and illness* (6th ed.). Upper Saddle River, NJ: Pearson Education.

Spector, R. E. (2004b). *Cultural care guide to heritage assessment and health traditions* (3rd ed.). Upper Saddle River, NJ: Pearson Prentice Hall.

Spector, R. E. (2009). *Cultural diversity in health and illness* (7th ed.). Upper Saddle River, NJ: Pearson Education.

Statue of Liberty–Ellis Island Foundation. (2010). *Ellis Island-history.* Retrieved February 14, 2011, from http://www.ellisisland.org/genealogy/ellis_island_history.asp

U.S. Department of Health and Human Services, Health Resources and Services Administration. (2010). *The registered nurse population: Initial findings from the 2008 national sample survey of registered nurses.* Retrieved February 2, 2011, from http://bhpr.hrsa.gov/healthworkforce/rnsurvey

NCLEX-TYPE TEST QUESTIONS (1–15)

1. While attending orientation, a newly hired nurse asks the certified transcultural nurse (CTN): "Is the language access services of the culturally and linguistically appropriate services (CLAS) mandatory for all institutions? Which of the following responses from the CTN is most appropriate?
   A. "Only institutions with a certain number of beds are mandated."
   B. "Only institutions receiving federal fundings are mandated."
   C. "Only institutions receiving private fundings are mandated."
   D. "Only institutions receiving state funding are mandated."

2. You are the nurse educator planning for orientation session for new nurses from India. In the area of social organization, which one of the following questions is most likely to obtain information?
   A. "How do you plan to manage homesickness?"
   B. "Do you plan to manage homesickness?"
   C. "Will you be planning to manage homesickness?"
   D. "Do you have a plan to manage homesickness?"

3. The operating room nurse is preparing a client with gastrointestinal bleeding for surgery. The nurse noticed an orange string tied around the client's wrist. Which of the following approaches is most culturally congruent?
   A. "I see that string on your wrist. May I remove it?"
   B. "I see that string on your wrist. Would you remove it?"
   C. "I see that string on your wrist. May I tape it in place?"
   D. "I see that string on your wrist. Would you mind removing it?"

4. The nurse is discharging a Haitian diabetic client who works as a migrant laborer for a farm nearby. The nurse observes that the client lowers his gaze instead of looking at her directly. Which of the following explanations is most appropriate?
   A. Avoidance of direct gaze is a sign of respect.
   B. Avoidance of direct gaze is a sign of disinterest.
   C. Avoidance of direct gaze is a sign of disrespect.
   D. Avoidance of direct gaze is a sign of lack of affect.

5. A Jewish client refuses to take a newly ordered medication in gelatin form. Which of the following is the most appropriate statement from the nurse?
   A. "How come you are not taking this medication? This is important to control your blood pressure."
   B. "You must have a reason for not taking this medication. This is important to control your blood pressure."
   C. "Any reason for not taking this medication? This is important to control your blood pressure."
   D. "Please explain the reason for not taking this medication. This is important to control your blood pressure."

6. Your Irish American client is 1-day postoperative for abdominal surgery. You noticed that he appears tense and restless but refuses the pain medication that you offered. Which one of the following statements is the most culturally congruent?
   A. "You need not be stoic; taking the medication before the pain becomes unbearable is a more effective way to control pain."
   B. "Taking the medication before the pain becomes unbearable is a more effective way to control pain."
   C. "You need the medication before the pain becomes unbearable; it is a more effective way to control pain."
   D. "Taking the medication before the pain becomes unbearable is a more correct way to control pain."

7. According to Spector, heritage consistency involves determining one's background in terms of:
   A. culture, ethnicity, and religion
   B. culture, language, and religion
   C. culture, ethnicity, and time orientation
   D. culture, space, and religion

8. Spector used which of the following authors' six cultural phenomena to develop the personal health tradition of a unique cultural being?
   A. Josepha Campinha-Bacote
   B. Purnell and Paulanka
   C. Leininger and McFarland
   D. Giger and Davidhizar

9. Which of the following responses by the instructor is the most therapeutic for a Navajo nursing student who appears reluctant to perform postmortem care on a client?
   A. "Although postmortem care is not a required competency, you must take the opprtunity as it arises."
   B. "This is optional experience and entirely dependent on your decision."
   C. "You seem distressed to perform postmortem care. Would you like to discuss it."
   D. "You seem distressed to perform postmortem care. I will send you home."

10. A new adjunct faculty member comes to the full-time faculty adviser of a Vietnamese American nursing student. The adjunct faculty said: "She was so distressed about her patient dying so I tried to pat her on the head. She jumped out of her skin it startled me; then she would not explain it." Which of the following statements is the most appropriate by the faculty adviser?
    A. "Vietnamese Americans believe that the head is sensitive and should not be touched unnecesarily by others."
    B. "Vietnamese Americans believe that the head is sacred and should not be touched unnecesarily by others."
    C. "Vietnamese Americans believe that the head is a private part and should not be touched unnecesarily by others."
    D. "Vietnamese Americans believe that the head is important and should not be touched unnecesarily by others."

11. According to Spector, which of the following is not an aspect of health in the traditional context?
    A. maintaining health
    B. protecting health
    C. restoring health
    D. promoting health

12. You are the faculty adviser to the Vietnamese Nursing Student Association at the university. The association's president invited you to tea at the association's first anniverary celebration. Which of the following questions is most important for you to ask?
    A. "What kind of food should I bring?"
    B. "What type of clothes or color should I wear?"
    C. "What type of shoes should I wear?"
    D. "What time should I arrive?"

13. The nurse is caring for a non-English speaking Lithuanian client who had gotten ill while visiting a relative in the United States. This morning, the patient is withdrawn, hostile, and uncooperative. According to Spector, this client may be experiencing:
    A. cultural shock
    B. socialization
    C. cultural imposition
    D. acculturation

14. The nurse is caring for a client from Thailand who has limited English proficiency. According to the culturally and linguistically appropriate services (CLAS) standards, this client:
    A. does not need an interpreter since he is able to speak some words of English
    B. does need an interpreter since he is able only to speak some words of English
    C. does need a translator since he is able only to speak some words of English
    D. does not need a translator since he is able to speak some words of English

15. The nurse is preparing to give a workshop on postpartum depression to a group of pregnant Mexican American women. Having reviewed evidence-based literature, she knows that which of the following is of utmost importance for Mexican Americans?
    A. punctuality
    B. persistence
    C. respect
    D. honesty

(Answers to these questions can be found on p. 145)

6

Margaret Andrews/Joyceen Boyle Transcultural Nursing Assessment Guide for Individuals and Families

SECTION 1. REVIEW OF THE GUIDE

Andrews and Boyle (2008) developed 12 categories of cultural knowledge that are not only vital in cultural and physical assessment but invaluable in developing culturally competent care for individuals, families, groups, communities, and institutions. The guide's major categories are:

- "cultural affiliations;
- values orientation;
- communication;
- health-related beliefs and practices;
- nutrition;
- socioeconomic considerations;
- organizations providing cultural support;
- education;
- religion;
- cultural aspects of disease incidence;
- biocultural variations; and
- developmental considerations across the life span" (Andrews & Boyle, 2008, p. 35).

The explicit addition of the life span component contributes to this guide's uniqueness among transcultural assessment tools. While there are other cultural assessment tools for individuals and families, the transcultural nursing assessment guide for individual and families (TCNAGIF) is among the few that contain features for community assessment (Boyle, 2008) and assessment for organizational cultural competence.

Nurse–patient interactions entail the interaction of three cultural systems (American Nurses Association [ANA], 1991). Andrews (2008b) developed a conceptual model for understanding cultural influences on nurse–client interactions (Figure 6.1). The model succinctly illustrates

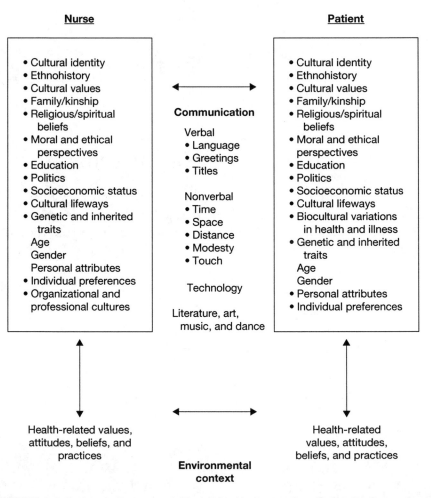

FIGURE 6.1 Andrews Conceptual Model for Understanding Cultural Influences on Nurse–Patient Interactions.

Source: Reprinted by permission from Andrews, M. M. (2008b). Culturally competent nursing care. In M. M. Andrews & J. S. Boyle (Eds.), *Transcultural concepts in nursing care* (5th ed., pp. 15–33). Philadelphia, PA: Wolters Kluwer/Lippincott Williams & Wilkins. Copyright Wolters Kluwer/Lippincott Williams & Wilkins.

the process of cross-cultural communications both verbally and non-verbally between the nurse and the patient and the family or significant other (Andrews, 2008b).

Emerging from a collaboration between faculty and doctoral students at the University of Utah, the initial publication of the book *Transcultural Concepts in Nursing Care* in 1989 aimed to clarify application of transcultural nursing (TCN) principles in clinical practice (Andrews & Boyle, 2002). The book received the American Journal of Nursing *Book of the Year Award* and Sigma Theta Tau International Honor Society of Nursing's *Best Pick Award*. This TCN textbook has been organized into four sections: foundation of TCN; developmental approach across the life span; application in nursing care delivery; and contemporary challenges in TCN. Believing that "a comprehensive cultural assessment is the foundation of culturally competent nursing care," Andrews and Boyle (2002, p. 179) recommended the use of the TCNAGIF to gather relevant data; they did not include any nursing care of a particular ethnic or cultural group. Now in its fifth edition, Andrews and Boyle's (2008) textbook is the one that nursing schools use (Boyle, 2007) to organize the curricula when they prefer not to use a specific TCN model (Lipson & Desantis, 2007).

Leininger's culture care diversity and universality (CCDU) theory and contribution to the development of TCN, along with theoretic concepts from natural and behavioral sciences, are thoroughly discussed in the foundation section. Notably, these are among a few of Dr. Leininger's achievements in the field of TCN: (1) noting and studying of differences in care (1954); (2) offering of telecourses in TCN and establishment of first PhD in anthropology and nursing, University of Colorado School of Nursing, Denver, CO (1965–1969); (3) founding of the first TCN academic department, University of Washington School of Nursing, Seattle, WA (1973); (4) establishment of *Transcultural Nursing Society* (TCNS) (1974); (5) founding and initiation of TCNS certification in TCN (CTN) (1988); and (6) publication of *Journal of Transcultural Nursing* (1989) (Andrews & Boyle, 2008). Leininger was also credited for the first TCN research, which she conducted in depth for 2 years among the Gadsups of the highlands of New Guinea (Andrews, 2006; Leininger & McFarland, 2006). The second section contains TCN concepts as they apply to the entire life span of child-bearing clients, children, adolescents, adults, and older age clients with some illustration of TCN issues, trends, and problems. In the third section, the textbook illustrates application of TCN in mental health, management of pain, community health nursing, and cultural aspects of families and communities (Andrews & Boyle, 2002, 2008). The fourth section highlights contemporary challenges in TCN including pain management;

religion, culture, and nursing; ethical decision making; and international nursing.

Fundamentally, the nurse needs to engage in his or her own cultural self-assessment and needs to be aware of his/her own values, attitudes, beliefs, and practices that have been handed down by the family from generation to generation (Andrews, 2008b). The cultural self-asessment will assist in overcoming biases, prejudices, and ethnocentrism. Andrews (2008b) emphasized that the cultural self-assessment is a prerequisite to cultural assessment of others. Leininger (2002b) warned that cultural blindness, the "inability to know another culture because of cultural biases, attitudes, and prejudices" (p. 122) may occur if the nurse does not engage in full self-assessment. Like Campinha-Bacote (2002, 2005a, 2007), Andrews and Boyle (2002, 2008) refer to cultural competence as a continuous process and not an end point.

SECTION 2. APPLICATION OF THE GUIDE IN NURSING EDUCATION

The transcultural assessment guide for individuals and families (Andrews & Boyle, 2002, 2008) offers a comprehensive guide for an assessment tool in undergraduate and graduate programs. The guide may also be used in physical assessment and other nursing courses in the master's programs. Moreover, components of the TCNAGIF such as biocultural variations and cultural aspects of the disease and nutrition, among others, will be appropriate for advanced courses in physical assessment, pharmacology, adult and geriatric health, maternal and child, child, and other nursing and health classes.

In their surveys of nursing programs to determine teaching and learning methods employed to foster knowledge, attitudes, and skills in cultural competence, Lipson and Desantis (2007) indicated that some of the schools build their courses around Andrews and Boyle's (2003) textbook. This textbook is also credited for adding to the evolution of TCN; its assessment tool vital to developing culturally competent care (Glittenberg, 2004). The organization of this textbook into (1) transcultural concepts, (2) developmental approach, (3) application of concepts in nursing care delivery, and (4) contemporary challenges (Andrews & Boyle, 2002) is systematic, holistic, and designed to improve health care of individuals, families, groups, and communities. Andrews and Boyle (2002) designed this book for introductory undergraduate TCN courses and as a reference for nurses who had no formal preparation in TCN. Moreover, Andrews and Boyle's strong commitment to theory development is evident in their use of Leininger's theoretic framework for TCN practice; they clarified that their guide is not a theory or conceptual model. Contained in *Transcultural Concepts in Nursing Care* are "clinical applications of TCN concepts, theories, and research across the life span and in a variety of health care settings" (Andrews & Boyle, 2002, p. 180).

The TCNAGIF by Andrews and Boyle (2002, 2008) may be applied to all programs in nursing education, from licensed practical to doctoral nursing programs. In Table 6.1, the TCNAGIF is used to guide an assignment to introduce cultural diversity and cultural competence among students in a licensed practical nursing (LPN) program who may have very little exposure to this area. Some LPN programs are offered in the senior year in high school; other programs require completion of high school and may vary in length from 8 months to a year.

TABLE 6.1 Application of the TAGIF in a NUR 1110—Introduction to Practical Nursing (2 Credits)

NUR 1110- Introduction to Practical Nursing (2 credits)
Prerequisites

Module 1. Communication
  1. Barriers to effective communication
    A. Non-English– or limited English proficiency–speaking patient
  2. Facilitators of effective communication
    B. Interpretation versus translation

Module 3. Kinship and social networks
  1. Patient's family and its role in health and illness
  2. Beliefs and healing practices
  3. Gender issues

Module 2. Nutrition
  1. Definition of food
  2. Cultural preferences, preparation, fasting
  3. Home and folk remedies

Assignment. Observe unit for clinical affiliation as you go for your rotation. List your answers to the folowing questions and be prepared to discuss during postconference starting on clinical day 5.
  1. How many nurses belong to each of the following ethnic groups: White, Hispanic, African American, Asian.
  2. How many students in your class belong to each of the following ethnic groups: White, Hispanic, African American, Asian.
  3. How many patients in this unit belong to each of the following ethnic groups: White, Hispanic, African American, Asian.
  4. Discuss some questions in your mind based on these observations.

In doctoral programs, the TCNAGIF may be used in core courses in the education, administration, or clinical tracts in preparation for a dissertation topic. Leininger's (2002a, 2006a; Leininger & McFarland, 2006) ethnonursing method would be an ideal choice of pursuing the student's topic of interest. Table 6.2 shows the application of TCNAGIF in a course in a doctoral program. The students may choose from the TCNAGIF; Leininger's CCDU; or any of the TCN models such as Campinha-Bacote's Biblically based model of cultural competence (2003a, 2005a); Giger and Davidhizar's (2004, 2008) transcultural assessment model; Purnell's (2008) Model for Cultural Competence; and Spector's (2004a, 2009) health traditions model. The faculty may also draw from a hat to ensure that all theory, models, and guide will be presented and studied in class. Each student presentation will cover the guidelines and integration of concepts in a licensed practical, associate or diploma, baccalaureate, and master's program.

TABLE 6.2 Application of the TAGIF in a Core Course at a Doctoral Program

NUR 6000-Transcultural Nursing Education	Credits-3	Prerequisites—Completion of a Master's Degree in Nursing

This course explores the integration of Transcultural Nursing (TCN) concepts and the promotion of cultural competence in nursing curricula using the Andrews/Boyle assessment for individuals and families (TCNAGIF). The student will develop creative means to explore how TCNAGIF could be actually threaded in the curricula of a licensed practical, an associate, a baccalaureate, and a master's program.

Guide

1. Literature review: Integration of TCN concepts in nursing curricula.
2. You may use existing curricular plans from the aforementioned programs. Show all revisions that you will develop. Be creative.
3. You may create a visionary curricula for every level of the programs above. Be creative.
4. Review the following audiovisual resources and determine what curricular level(s) you would integrate. Please provide your rationales.
    4.1. Grainger-Monsen, M., & Haslett, J. (2003). *Words apart: A four-part series on cross cultural healthcare.* Boston, MA: Fanlight Production.
    Mohammad Kochi's story: Afghanistan
    Justine Chitsena's story: Khmu from Laos
    Robert Philips' story: African American
    Alicia Mercado's story: Puerto Rico
    4.2 Boise State University Department of Nursing. (2007). *Dialogues in culture.* Boise, ID: Author.
    Dialogue on refugees
    Dialogue on Iraq war veterans
    Dialogue on Native Americans
    Dialogue on the lesbian, gay, bisexual, and transgender community
    4.3 Are there other audiovisual resources that you could use?

For nurse educators in staff development, there is an ever-present challenge of reaching staff nurses from all shifts. If the hospital or agency uses the TCNAGIF as its framework to integrate cultural diversity and promote cultural competence, the nurse educator could use posters in the unit or where nurses take their break times. A copy of Andrews and Boyle's *Transcultural Concepts in Nursing Care* (2008) needs to be available on every unit and at the library. Copy of the TCNAGIF needs to be in every unit posted at strategic places. Lunch meetings or "brown bag meetings" could be a mutually available time to discuss important areas of accreditation standards that call for cultural competence as well as research and evidence-based practice (EBP) that improve patient outcomes. Strategies like this have been used to promote evidence-based practice in general. In addition, requiring additional time on the part of the nurses will spark resistance, so release time is important (DiCenso, Guyatt, & Ciliska, 2005; Polit & Beck, 2010). Release time for EBP will become part of the organizational plan if there is commitment on the part of the nursing administration (Polit & Beck, 2010). Awarding of continuing education (CE) credits promotes attendance; CE is seen as a reward for lifelong learning or as an incentive for maintaining registration for continued licensure or toward specialty certification requirements.

SECTION 3. APPLICATION OF THE GUIDE IN NURSING PRACTICE

Cultural assessment has been defined as the "systematic, comprehensive examination of individuals, families, groups, and communities regarding their health-related cultural beliefs, values, and practices" (Andrews & Boyle, 2008, p. 34). The cultural assessment is vital in determining health care needs and planning meaningful and culturally congruent care (Leininger & McFarland, 2006). Leininger (2002b) enumerated several purposes of the culture care assessment of clients: (1) health patterns and meanings, (2) holistic information, (3) potential areas of conflicts and clashes, (4) general and specific themes, and (5) similarities and differences (p. 119). The two important components of the cultural assessment are the transcultural perspectives in health history and perspectives in the physical examination (Andrews, 2008a). The TCNAGIF is a tool that is meant to hone the nurse's assessment skills; when used along with critical thinking, the nurse will be able to render culturally competent care (Andrews & Boyle, 2008).

When the nurse has completed the health history and physical examination, an analyis of the subjective and objective data, and mutual goal setting with the client, she may use any or all of the three modalities of action in order to provide culturally congruent care: cultural preservation or maintenance; cultural care accomodation or negotiation; and cultural repatterning or restructuring (Andrews, 2008a; Leininger, 2002b; Leininger & McFarland, 2006).

The TCNAGIF is highly applicable in many practice settings. For example, in community health nursing, it could be used as a guide for assessment, planning, interventions, and evaluations of nursing care. As hospitalization days get shorter and clients are discharged much earlier and back to the community, there are challenges for community health nurses. Nurses work in various community settings such as department of health, schools, clinics, and the client's home. In home care, nurses are in that unique position to assess the client and family or significant other in their own environment. It becomes imperative that the nurse understand family values, lifestyle, health practices including the cultural determinants of behavior related to health and illness (Boyle, 2008). Some clients have lifelong illnesses; it is vital that the nurse include culturally congruent care to motivate clients' behavior modifications for better outcomes. Focusing on the community as client is the thrust of community-based nursing (Stanhope & Lancaster, 2010). Culturally competent care has the potential of improving the health of the community, including those at higher risk such as the poor, and the homeless, and those with human immunodeficiency virus, acquired immunodeficiency syndrome, and/or tuberculosis (Andrews, 2008b; Boyle, 2008; Stanhope & Lancaster, 2010). According to Boyle (2008), using the epidemiologic and transcultural model—by identifying three aspects: (1) subcultures and planning community-based interventions, (2) various components of the community, and (3) values and cultural norms (pp. 264–265)—enhances nurse community interactions, which are essential in implementing appropriate interventions.

When selecting cultural research for EBP, it is important not to rely solely on quantitative studies that may show *how effective a medication is* but to use qualitative studies where there may be culturally based answers as to *why clients refuse to take the medications based on preferences and values* (Polit & Beck, 2010). There is an accumulation of research done with the use of the ethnonursing method, founded and initiated by Leininger in the early 1960s with her 2-year research about the Gadsup people in New Guinea, to the current era (Andrews, 2006,

2008b; Leininger, 2006a; Leininger & McFarland, 2006), generating over 400 studies before the year 2000 (Glittenberg, 2004). Categories from Andrews and Boyle's (2002, 2008) TCNAGIF such as communication, values orientation, health-related beliefs and practices, nutrition, and socioeconomic considerations are assessment areas that are applicable in this situation.

Whether planning health education for an individual, individuals and families, communities, or organizations, the TCNAGIF (Andrews & Boyle, 2002, 2008) may easily be applied. Table 6.3 shows its application in the care of Mr. Trinh, a 70-year-old Vietnamese American client.

TABLE 6.3 Components of Andrews and Boyle Transcultural Assessment Guide Applied to the Care of Vietnamese American Client

Components	Assessment	Nursing Interventions and Rationales
Biocultural variations and cultural aspects of the incidence of disease	Lactose intolerance is prevalent	1. Substitute soy milk, beans, etc., for milk and other dairy products
Communication	Understands a few English words. Originally from South Vietnam	1. Use language access services (determine dialect first) for either face-to-face or remote interpretation
Cultural affiliations	Goes to senior citizen group comprising Vietnamese and Filipino members	1. Encourage to go back to the group after discharge
Cultural sanctions and restrictions	The head is considered sacred and should not be touched unnecessarily	1. Explain necessary procedures such as assessment, etc 2. Assess for expressions of pain
Developmental considerations	Task is integrity versus despair (Erikson, 1968 as cited in Schwecke, 2003)	1. Allow expressions of life stories
Economics	Came by boat as a refugee. Spent 6 months at a camp in Thailand. Medicaid pending	1. Refer to social worker and counseling; if possible to bilingual practitioners; if not use interpreter
Educational background	Sixth grade education	1. Ensure that teaching is simple; patient education materials are at that level
Health-related beliefs and practices	Home remedies first, relies on folk medicine	1. Has bruising on back along riblines; assess for other remedies

(Continued)

TABLE 6.3 *Continued*

Components	Assessment	Nursing Interventions and Rationales
Kinship and social networks	Family is very important; has a large extended family	1. Allow family to visit; take turns
Nutrition	Strictly vegetarian	1. Allow family to bring food from home; teach diet restriction if any
		2. Consult with pharmacy about ingredients in medications in capsule form; make sure insulin is not from pork or beef sources
Religion and spirituality	Practicing Buddhist	1. Inform availability of hospital nondenominational temple
Values orientation	Respect is very important	1. Be respectful at all times; address as Mr. Trinh

Source: Developed from M. M. Andrews & J. S. Boyle. (2008). *Transcultural concepts in nursing care* (5th ed.). Philadelphia, PA: Wolters Kluwer Lippincott, Williams, & Wilkins; Sagar, P. L. (2000). *The lived experience of Vietnamese nurses: A case study.* Ed.D. dissertation, Columbia University Teachers College, New York. Retrieved January 28, 2011, from ProQuest Dissertations & Theses. (Publication No. AAT 9959348); Wenger, F. A. (2006). Culture care and health of Russian and Vietnamese refugee communities in the United States. In M. Leininger & M. McFarland (Eds.), *Transcultural nursing: Concepts, theories, research, and practice* (3rd ed., pp. 327–348). New York, NY: McGraw-Hill Companies.

SECTION 4. APPLICATION OF THE GUIDE IN NURSING ADMINISTRATION

Andrews and Boyle (2002, 2008) had firmly explicated that neither their guide nor their textbook is a theory nor a framework of TCN; they base their work on Leininger's theory. The CCDU has been applied in two chapters of Andrews and Boyle's (2008) about nursing administration and about nursing in a multicultural health care setting. Leininger (2002c) refers to TCN administration as "the creative and knowledgeable process of assessing, planning, and making decisions and policies that will facilitate educational and clinical service goals that take into account caring values, beliefs, symbols, and lifeways of people of diverse cultures for beneficial outcomes" (p. 563). Andrews (2008c) voiced the need for nurse administrators to acknowledge the basic value system embraced by staff in order to understand their behavior. Selected components of TCNAGIF (Andrews & Boyle, 2008) such as communication, cultural affiliations, developmental considerations, educational background, and values orientation will be important to assess when making decisions about cost benefit outcome, downsizing, and other contemporary challenges in administering a complex, multicultural workplace.

Maintaining that transcultural theoretic knowledge and skills are imperative in guiding administrators as advocates for change, Hubbert (2006) specified the applicability of Leininger's CCDU for nurse administrators and managers. Nurse administrators are directly involved in the globalization of health care and should have the necessary skills for team building in the ever-changing and complex system (Hubbert, 2006). To be an effective administrator and manager, one has to be cognizant of the three culture systems in nurse–client interactions: "the culture of the nurse, the culture of the client, and the culture of the setting" (ANA, 1991, para 7). Nurse administrators and managers are expected to function within these diverse cultures and subcultures and facilitate culturally congruent care (Hubbert, 2006; Leininger, 2006b).

In a culturally competent organization, Ludwig-Beymer (2008) quoted: "health care services are respectful of and responsive to the cultural and linguistic needs of patients" (p. 198). Ludwig-Beymer also outlined the process of creating a culturally competent organization using assessment tools such as Leininger's (2002a, 2006a) CCDU and the forces of magnetism by the American Nurses Credentialing Center (2005). Cognizant of the three culture system interactions, Ludwig-Beymer (2008) encouraged administrators to integrate Leininger's (2002a, 2002c, 2002d, 2006a) three action modes in ensuring that culturally sensitive organizational policies are in place. In addition, Ludwig-Beymer (2008) cited Malone's 1997 strategies for enhancing organizational competence: implementing training that values and manages diversity; rewarding collaborative practice that celebrates differences; seeking culturally competent members; and recruiting and hiring culturally diverse members. Andrews (2008c) likewise constructed a set of guidelines in performing both a cultural assessment of individuals and organizations.

Clinical and academic administrators of the future will need graduate preparation in TCN (Leininger, 2002c, 2006b). While many administrators now are focused on preparing nurse practitioners for cost-effective care, it is noteworthy to point out that nurse administrators and staff with graduate preparation in TCN can be cost-effective and able to promote health and expedite recovery from illness (Leininger, 2002c, 2006b).

There are conflicting numbers of non-English speakers in the United States; the figures lay between 12% and 19% of the population or as many as 52 million people aged 5 years and older (Andrews & Boyle, 2008; Berry-Caban & Crespo, 2008). The Sullivan Commission (2004) reported that 2 out of 10 Americans speak a language other than English at home. Twelve to 19% of the population is an alarming number and a huge concern—considering that language is vital in access and quality of health care (Stanhope & Lancaster, 2010) and is frequently mentioned as the primary barrier to health care (Berry-Caban & Crespo, 2008). Communication between providers and clients must indeed be a priority for nurse administrators and managers.

On the one hand are clients who speak English as a second language (ESL) or have limited English proficiency (LEP)—on the other could be health care workers who also speak ESL—this could contribute to other communication problems. Problems in communication in the multicultural workplace arise with different languages and accents. Telephonic communication may intensify this problem (Andrews, 2008c); an example of this would be receiving and giving orders by phone. When planning orientation for foreign nurses, the area of communication is as important as infection control and other annual mandates for staff development.

Nurse administrators must ensure that the organization is in compliance not only with culturally and linguistically appropriate services (CLAS) standards, but will need to widely disseminate The Joint Commission (TJC) resources: *Cultural Sensitivity: A Pocket Guide for Health Care Professionals* (Galanti & Woods, 2007), *Advancing Effective Communication, Cultural Competence, and Patient- and Family-Centered Care: A Roadmap for Hospitals* (TJC, 2010a), and *Cultural and Linguistic Care in Area Hospitals* (TJC, 2010b). Galanti and Woods (2007) developed a pocket guide that contains core cultural patterns such as (1) values, worldview, and communication; (2) family/gender issues; (3) cradle to grave practices; and (4) health-related beliefs and practices for clients who are African Americans/Anglo American; Asian; Hispanic/Latino; Jewish; Middle Eastern; Native American; Russian; South Asian; and Southeast Asian. TJC (2010a) calls upon the buy-in and support from hospital administration and leaders in communicating leadership commitment to "effective communication, cultural competence, and patient- and family-centered care," "in engaging staff regularly and ongoing basis, in assigning individuals accountable to leadership to advance this initiatives, and in integrating the CLAS into the hospital services, programs, and initiatives" (p. 34). Appendix C shows an example of CE workshop for health care workers that integrate CLAS and other important areas for cultural competency training of health care workers.

TJC (2010b) conducted a study of 14 hospitals in Florida regarding the availability of cultural and linguistic resources and services at each hospital. Through purposive sampling, TJC (2010b) collected data with two questionnaires: (1) availability of cultural and linguistic services, and (2) staff awareness of services, staff use of services, and staff reason for use of services. Findings indicate that all hospitals provide varied tools, resources, and services to meet clients' cultural and linguistic needs (TJC, 2010b). Furthermore, TJC (2010b) results specified that the staff were not always aware of services; if there is staff awareness, the staff did not frequently use the services; and staff "still use someone accompanying the patient" (p. 34). The study did not ask the staff to evaluate the services nor investigate the effectiveness of the tools and resources being used. It appears that this gap in knowledge from provider and client standpoints are areas of future research in order not only to quantify the effectiveness of such tools and resources but also to explore the satisfaction of clients and families using the resources.

Case Scenario

This scenario involves the chief executive officer (CEO), director of nursing (DON), nurse manager and the registered nurse (RN) at Sunrise Hospital, and a 200-bed community hospital in the western part of the United States. Ninety percent of the population in the area are White. There is a large influx of Mexican immigrants in the last 20 years; this population accounts for about 8% of the total population. The remaining segment of the population are Native Americans. The emergency department (ED) is newly refurbished from a grant and is tasefully decorated with paintings that depict the settling of the west. None of the pictures show any Native or Mexican Americans. Modern and comfortable furnitures and rugs do not include any design of Native or Mexican American origins. Although there is some signage in Spanish, they are neither at strategic places nor in fonts that are easily visible.

DON: (Dressed in a suit) The DON is visibly upset, having had a meeting with the CEO who had narrated a complaint from the son of a previous ED client. The client is 73 years old, has congestive heart failure, lives alone, and has LEP. The client's son complained about the care his father received in the ED. The client, having been initially taken to the ED by ambulance for severe shortness of breath, was not offered an interpreter. The client later told his son that he did not want to upset his granddaughter so he did not narrate how sick he actually was.

Nurse manager of ED: She explains that the RN is a new graduate and only started at the hospital 9 months ago. The RN was really busy that night and had instead used, as interpreter, the client's 20-year-old granddaughter who arrived shortly after her grandfather's admission to the ED. In the RN's haste, he forgot to explain the availability of interpreters at no extra cost to the client. The RN did admit to the nurse manager that he remembers something about standards for language access that he had during his 2-week orientation to the hospital. During his 2-week preceptorship, he does not recall any situation about using interpreters since his previous Mexican immigrant patients "can speak passable English and always come in with an entourage of family members."

Transcultural nurse (CTN-A): Dressed in a laboratory coat. He/she will act as the facilitator and moderate the discussion following the role playing. Some suggested guide questions are as follow:

1. How is communication as a component of the TCNAGIF involved here? What other components of the TCNAGIF could you include? Discuss. Why is it important to use existing theory, models, and guide with current federal, accreditation, and other relevant guidelines?
2. How are these three documents, namely, *Advancing Effective Communication, Cultural Competence, and Patient- and Family-Centered Care: A Roadmap for Hospitals* and *Cultural and Linguistic Care in Area Hospitals* (TJC, 2010a, 2010b) and the *Culturally and Linguistically Appropriate Service*s standards (U.S. Department of Health and Human Services, Office of Minority Health, 2001) vital in this scenario? Discuss.
3. Would you include salient points from the aforementioned documents, along with TJC-specific standards for improvement at your institution, at staff meetings at all levels, and in yearly competencies? Discuss.
4. How would you design the ED to make it more welcoming to the Native American members of this community?
5. Reenact the scenario.

Instructor/Educator: Debriefing

1. Reflect on the role play. How did you feel?
2. Discuss what you learned. What other learning needs do you have? Discuss.
3. Discuss the clinical application of this role play.

4. Examine the changes needed in your own knowledge, skills, and behavior in order to incorporate culturally congruent care in nursing education, practice, and administration.

REFERENCES

American Nurses Association. (1991). *Position statement on cultural diversity in nursing practice.* Kansas City, MO: Author.

American Nurses Credentialing Center. (2005). *Magnet recognition program: Recognizing excellence in nursing service.* Silver Springs, MD: Author.

Andrews, M. M. (2006). The globalization of transcultural nursing theory and research. In M. M. Leininger & M. R. McFarland (Eds.), *Culture care diversity and universality: A worldwide nursing theory* (2nd ed., pp. 83–114). Sudbury, MA: Jones & Bartlett.

Andrews, M. M. (2008a). Cultural competence in the health history and physical examination. In M. M. Andrews & J. S. Boyle (Eds.), *Transcultural concepts in nursing care* (5th ed., pp. 34–65). Philadelphia, PA: Wolters Kluwer/Lippincott Williams & Wilkins.

Andrews, M. M. (2008b). Culturally competent nursing care. In M. M Andrews & J. S. Boyle (Eds.), *Transcultural concepts in nursing care* (5th ed., pp. 15–33). Philadelphia, PA: Wolters Kluwer/Lippincott Williams & Wilkins.

Andrews, M. M. (2008c). Cultural diversity in the health care workforce. In M. M. Andrews & J. S. Boyle (Eds.), *Transcultural concepts in nursing care* (5th ed., pp. 297–326). Philadelphia, PA: Wolters Kluwer/Lippincott Williams & Wilkins.

Andrews, M. M., & Boyle, J. S. (2002). Transcultural concepts in nursing care. *Journal of Transcultural Nursing, 13*(3), 178–180.

Andrews, M. M., & Boyle, J. S. (2008). Andrews/Boyle transcultural nursing assessment guide for individuals and families. In M. M. Andrews & J. S. Boyle (Eds.), *Transcultural concepts in nursing care* (5th ed., pp. 453–460). Philadelphia, PA: Wolters Kluwer/Lippincott Williams & Wilkins.

Andrews, M. M., & Boyle, J. S. (2008). *Transcultural concepts in nursing care* (5th ed.). Philadelphia, PA: Wolters Kluwer/Lippincott Williams & Wilkins.

Berry-Caban, C. S., & Crespo, H. (2008). Cultural competency as a skill for health care providers. *Hispanic Health International, 6*(3), 115–121.

Boise State University Department of Nursing. (2007). *Dialogues in culture.* Boise, ID: Author.

Boyle, J. (2007). Commentary on "Current approaches to integrating elements of cultural competence in nursing education." *Journal of Transcultural Nursing, 18*(1), 21S–22S.

Boyle, J. S. (2008). Culture, family and community. In M. M. Andrews & J. S. Boyle (Eds.), *Transcultural concepts in nursing care* (5th ed., pp. 261–296). Philadelphia, PA: Wolters Kluwer/Lippincott Williams & Wilkins.

Campinha-Bacote, J. (2002). The process cultural competence in the delivery of healthcare services: A model of care. *Journal of Transcultural Nursing, 13*(3), 181–184.

Campinha-Bacote, J. (2003a). *The process cultural competence in the delivery of healthcare services: A Culturally competent model of care.* Cincinnati, OH: Transcultural C.A.R.E Associates.

Campinha-Bacote, J. (2005a). *A Biblically based model of cultural competence in the delivery of healthcare services.* Cincinnati, OH: Transcultural C.A.R.E Associates.

Campinha-Bacote, J. (2007). *The process cultural competence in the delivery of healthcare services: The journey continues.* Cincinnati, OH: Transcultural C.A.R.E Associates.

DiCenso, A., Guyatt, G., & Ciliska, D. (2005). *Evidence-based nursing: A guide to clinical practice.* St. Louis: MO: Elsevier Mosby.

Galanti, G., & Woods, M. (2007). *Cultural sensitvity: A pocket guide for health care professionals.* Oakbrook, IL: Joint Commission Resources.

Giger, J. N., & Davidhizar, R. E. (2004). *Transcultural nursing: Assessment and intervention* (4th ed.). St. Louis, MO: Mosby Elsevier.

Giger, J. N., & Davidhizar, R. E. (2008). *Transcultural nursing: Assessment and intervention.* (5th ed.). St. Louis, MO: Mosby Elsevier.

Glittenberg, J. (2004). A transdisciplinary, transcultural model for health care. *Journal of Transcultural Nursing, 15*(1), 6–10.

Grainger-Monsen, M., & Haslett, J. (2003). *Words apart: A four-part series on cross cultural healthcare.* Boston, MA: Fanlight Production.

Hubbert, A. (2006). Application of culture care theory for clinical nurse administrators and managers. In M. Leininger & M. McFarland (Eds.), *Culture care diversity and universality: A worldwide nursing theory* (pp. 349–364). Boston, MA: Jones & Bartlett.

Leininger, M. M. (2002a). Culture care theory: A major contribution to advance transcultural nursing knowledge and practices. *Journal of Transcultural Nursing, 13*(3), 189–192.

Leininger, M. M. (2002b). Culture care assessments for congruent competency practice. In M. Leininger & M. McFarland (Eds.), *Transcultural nursing: Concepts, theories, research, and practice* (3rd ed., pp. 117–143). New York, NY: McGraw-Hill Companies.

Leininger, M. M. (2002c). Transcultural nursing administration and consultation. In M. Leininger & M. McFarland (Eds.), *Transcultural nursing: Concepts, theories, research, and practice* (3rd ed., pp. 563–573). New York, NY: McGraw-Hill Companies.

Leininger, M. M. (2002d). Cultures and tribes of nursing, hospitals, and the medical culture. In M. Leininger & M. McFarland (Eds.), *Transcultural nursing: Concepts, theories, research, and practice* (3rd ed., pp. 181–204). New York, NY: McGraw-Hill Companies.

Leininger, M. M. (2006a). Culture care diversity and universality and evolution of the ethnonursing method. In M. Leininger & M. McFarland (Eds.), *Culture care diversity and universality: A worldwide nursing theory* (pp. 1–41). Boston, MA: Jones & Bartlett.

Leininger, M. M. (2006b). Culture care theory and uses in nursing administration. In M. Leininger & M. McFarland (Eds.), *Culture care diversity and universality: A worldwide nursing theory* (pp. 365–379). Boston, MA: Jones & Bartlett.

Leininger, M. M., & McFarland, M. R. (2006). *Culture care diversity and universality: A worldwide nursing theory.* Boston, MA: Jones & Bartlett.

Lipson, J. G., & Desantis, L. A. (2007). Current approaches to integrating elements of cultural competence in nursing education. *Journal of Transcultural Nursing, 18*(1), 10S–20S.

Ludwig-Beymer, P. (2008). Creating culturally competent organizations. In M. M. Andrews & J. S. Boyle (Eds.), *Transcultural concepts in nursing* (5th ed., pp. 197–225). Philadelphia, PA: Wolters Kluwer Health/Lippincott, Williams, & Wilkins.

Polit, D. F., & Beck, C. T. (2010). *Essentials of nursing research: Appraising evidence for nursing practice* (7th ed.). Philadelphia, PA: Wolters Kluwer/Lippincott, Williams, & Wilkins.

Purnell, L. D. (2008). The Purnell Model for cultural competence. In L. D. Purnel & B. J. Paulanka (Eds.), *Transcultural health care: A Culturally competent approach* (3rd ed., pp. 19–55). Philadelphia, PA: FA Davis.

Sagar, P. L. (2000). *The lived experience of Vietnamese nurses: A case study.* Ed.D. dissertation (Publication No. AAT 9959348). New York, NY: Columbia University Teachers College. Retrieved January 28, 2011, from ProQuest Dissertations & Theses.

Schwecke, L. H. (2003). Models for working with psychiatric patients. In L. N. Keltner, L. H. Schwecke, & C. E. Bostrom (Eds.), *Psychiatric Nursing* (4th ed., pp. 20–35). St. Louis, MO: Mosby/Elsevier.

Spector, R. E. (2004a). *Cultural diversity in health and illness* (6th ed.). Upper Saddle River, NJ: Pearson Education.

Spector, R. E. (2009). *Cultural diversity in health and illness* (7th ed.). Upper Saddle River, NJ: Pearson Education.

Stanhope, M., & Lancaster, J. (2010). *Foundations of nursing in the community: Community-oriented practice* (3rd ed.). St. Louis, MO: Mosby/Elsevier.

Sullivan Commission. (2004). *Missing persons: Minorities in the health professions: A report of the Sullivan Commission on diversity in the health care workforce.* Retrieved January 26, 2011, from www.jointcenter.org/healthpolicy/docs/Sullivan.pdf

The Joint Commission. (2010a). *Advancing effective communication, cultural competence, and patient- and family-centered care: A roadmap for hospitals.* Oakbrook Terrace, IL: Author.

The Joint Commission. (2010b). *Cultural and linguistic care in area hospitals.* Oakbrook Terrace, IL: Author.

U.S. Department of Health and Human Services, Office of Minority Health. (2001). *Culturally and linguistically appropriate services.* Retrieved August 26, 2011 from http://www.hhs.gov

Wenger, F. A. (2006). Culture care and health of Russian and Vietnamese refugee communities in the United States. In M. Leininger & M. McFarland (Eds.), *Transcultural nursing: Concepts, theories, research, and practice* (3rd ed., pp. 327–348). New York, NY: McGraw-Hill Companies.

NCLEX-TYPE TEST QUESTIONS (1–16)

1. Which of the following best describes the purpose of the Andrews and Boyle transcultural assessment for individuals and families?
   A. to contribute to the development of theoretically based transcultural nursing (TCN) and the advancement of TCN practice
   B. to analyze major issues encountered by nurses in providing TCN to individuals, families, groups, and communities
   C. to apply TCN framework to guide nursing practice in diverse health care settings
   D. to apply life span framework to guide nursing practice in diverse health care settings

2. In the process of client assessment, the nurse asks: "Are there healing rituals that you believe will hasten your recovery from illness?" The nurse is assessing which of the following areas of the Andrews and Boyle assessment guide?
   A. values orientation
   B. religion and spirituality
   C. kinship and social networks
   D. communication

3. The nurse is caring for a client with limited English proficiency and is in the process of selecting from a list of available trained interpreters. Which of the following questions is not applicable when selecting an interpreter for a client?
   A. Does the institution have available trained interpreters?
   B. Who would the client prefer to assist with interpretation?
   C. Is there anyone whom the client would prefer not to serve as interpreter?
   D. If there is no one available, could I use someone from housekeeping?

4. The nurse is validating assessment findings on the database of a 70-year-old Jewish patient on home care as she plans for additional help. The nurse asks: "Would you have any special request in terms of utensils for meals?" The nurse is assessing which of the following areas of the Andrews and Boyle assessment guide?
   A. values orientation
   B. religion and spirituality
   C. nutrition
   D. communication

5. The nurse is caring for a client who had migrated from Nigeria. Which one of the following questions would be more likely to elicit the client's cultural affiliation?
   A. Is African American your preferred cultural affiliation?
   B. What is the preferred term for your cultural affiliation?
   C. What is your cultural affiliation?
   D. Is Nigerian American your preferred cultural affiliation?

6. The pediatric nurse practitioner (PNP) is performing physical assessment of a 7-year-old Cambodian American boy. The boy's mother asks: "What should I do, he eats well but he has been small for his age?" Which of the following is the most appropriate response by the PNP?
   A. "He is not that small. Do not worry."
   B. "He is below the grid but the norming was done on Caucasian children."
   C. "He is not that small. He will grow and catch up. Do not worry."
   D. "He is below the grid but will be able to catch up. Do not worry."

7. The nurse educator at the Department of Health is using Andrews and Boyle's transcultural assessment guide in the orientation for new community health nurses. This guide is designed for:
   A. individuals and families only
   B. individuals, families, and groups
   C. individuals, families, groups, and communities
   D. individuals, families, groups, and aggregates

8. In all editions of the Andrews and Boyle's *Transcultural Concepts in Nursing*, the book is organized around which of the following areas?
   A. historical and theoretic foundations, multicultural health care settings, developmental approach, challenges
   B. historical and theoretic foundations, cultural groups, developmental approach, challenges
   C. historical and theoretic foundations, cultural and ethnic groups, developmental approach
   D. historical and theoretic foundations, multicultural groups, developmental approach, challenges

9. The nurse is performing physical examination of a dark-skinned client. To assess for jaundice, the nurse will check the client's:
   A. conjunctivae
   B. sclera
   C. oral mucosa
   D. earlobe

10. You are the nurse caring for a hypertensive Chinese American client who admitted to using ginseng for arthritic pain. The client added: "I use herbs only; but no medications." This situation is consistent with which of the following:
    A. Chinese Americans who use inhalant herbs do not consider herbs as drugs
    B. Chinese Americans who use oral herbs do not consider herbs as drugs
    C. Chinese Americans who smoke herbs do not consider herbs as drugs
    D. Chinese Americans who use topical herbs do not consider herbs as drugs

11. You are caring for a hypertensive Chinese American client who admitted to using ginseng for arthritic pain. You are very concerned because ginseng:
    A. potentiates antihypertensive drugs
    B. lowers blood pressure
    C. promotes youthful appearance
    D. increases longevity

12. In the process of assessing the effectiveness of her interventions, the nurse asks her non-English speaking client: "During the process of medical interpretation, did you feel that your wishes were honored and your needs communicated well?" The phase of the nursing process that the nurse is engaging is:
    A. evaluation
    B. assessment
    C. planning
    D. implementation

13. The non-English speaking client remarked to her daughter who in turn explained it to the nurse: "I do not have money to pay for an interpreter!" Which one of the following statements is the most accurate response by the nurse?
    A. "The language access services or medical interpretation is provided at a minimum cost to the patient."

B. "The language access services or medical interpretation is provided at moderate cost to the patient."

C. "The language access services or medical interpretation is provided at no extra cost to the patient."

D. "The language access services or medical interpretation is provided at little cost to the patient."

14. The sophomore student nurse heard the nurses referring to her assigned patient as "the Native American in room 216" while she noted that the nurses' aides refer to the client as "honey" or "grandpa." Which one of the following questions is most culturally sensitive for the student nurse to ask?
    A. "How would you prefer to be addressed?"
    B. "Would it be okay to call you grandpa?"
    C. "Would it be okay to call you honey?"
    D. "Would it be okay to call you Charles Littlejohn?"

15. While planning care for the mostly Filipino American children in the elementary school district, the family nurse practitioner (FNP) asks herself, "Are there any distinct growth and development characteristics among these children?" The FNP is assessing which one area of Andrews and Boyle's transcultural assessment guide?
    A. cultural affiliations
    B. developmental considerations
    C. health-related beliefs and practices
    D. cultural sanctions and restrictions

16. Your Haitian American client remarked to you as you were performing admission assessment: "I did not get sick because of any germs." Which one of the following assessment questions will be more culturally competent?
    A. "Please tell me then to what you believe caused your illness."
    B. "Tell me then what you think caused your illness."
    C. "Please tell me then what caused your illness."
    D. "Do tell me then to what cause you attribute your illness."

    (Answers to these questions can be found on p. 146)

7

DISCUSSION ACROSS MODELS AND FUTURE OF TRANSCULTURAL NURSING

SECTION 1. ACROSS THEORY, MODELS, AND GUIDE: WHERE ARE WE GOING?

This author reviewed one theory, five models, and one cultural assessment guide and explored a variety of ways to apply each one in nursing education, practice, and administration. The review is by no means exhaustive, but an attempt to include salient aspects of each as a guide in its limitless possibilities of applications in a variety of clinical settings of care, in academia, and in organizations. The reader is encouraged to return to the theory, models, and guide for details that may have been missed or concepts that have not been mentioned. This author concludes that the theory, models, and guide reviewed are all holistic. Health care providers—trained from empirics and rationality tend to lack holistic approach—tending to separate mind and body and may see clients as separate from the family or community (Berry-Caban & Crespo, 2008). The use of holistic models and guide will make the difference in the assessment, planning, and implementation, and evaluation of culturally congruent care.

The focus of this last part is to explore the usefulness of the theory, models, and guide into the current situations in health care and the implications in nursing education, nursing practice, and nursing administration. In the previous chapters, application of transcultural nursing (TCN) concepts in these settings has been explored with the use of scenarios, role plays, and tables.

On the occasion of the Transcultural Nursing Society (TCNS) International Conference in October 2001, the preconference symposium highlighted presentations from Drs. Leininger, Andrews and Boyle, Campinha-Bacote, Giger and Davidhizar, Purnell, and Spector. The presenters expounded on the evolution of their theory, models, and guide, and the respective clinical usefulness of each (Douglas, 2002). That gathering together of the authors of TCN theory, models, and guide had been 10 years ago. It is again time to reconvene and to continue to foster dialogue on the evolution of each theory, model, and guide. It is also time to include other TCN theory and models that may have been developed, used, and tested in that span of 10 years. Evaluation of each theory, model, and guide with criteria such as "congruence, inclusivity, scope, utility...." (Douglas, 2002, p. 177) could be revisited, adding other currently relevant criteria. As with cultures, the focus of this last part is to explore the applicability of each theory, models, and guide in the current situations in health care and the implications in nursing education, nursing practice, and nursing administration.

While it takes 8 to 15 years for a theory or new knowledge to be used in practice (Dobbins, Ciliska, Estabrooks, & Hayward, 2005), the ground is fertile for the application of new knowledge from the research using the culture care diversity and universality (CCDU) theory, the TCN models of Campinha-Bacote, Giger and Davidhizar, Purnell and Spector models, and the Andrews and Boyle transcultural nursing assessment guide for individuals and families in the areas of nursing education, practice, and administration. The awareness of current regulations, mandates, and guidelines are clarion calls to change from trickling to regular flow of TCN knowledge into teaching students; into enriching practice to care for diverse patients; into leading and managing increasingly complex organizations; and into urging necessary research in areas of disparities in access and quality of care and other gaps in knowledge. This awareness calls for application of cultural knowledge that lay dormant for many years despite laborious efforts from Dr. Leininger and those who have followed her path. Because of her ethnonursing method, research studies were conducted in areas too many to mention here and had produced results to enrich the enlarging body of knowledge in TCN (Andrews, 2006, 2008b; Glittenberg, 2004; Leininger & McFarland, 2006; McFarland, & Leininger, 2002; Ryan, 2011). Most of the visions and predictions of Dr. Leininger about the globalization of TCN and its worldwide impact had passed and will pass. Leininger predicted this as *The Third Era: Establishing Transcultural Nursing Worldwide* (Andrews, 2006; Leininger, 2002c; Leininger & McFarland, 2006).

SECTION 2. NURSING EDUCATION

Historically, the integration of cultural diversity in the nursing curricula is not new. In 1917, the National League for Nursing (NLN) Committee on Curriculum initially published a guide inclusive of sociology and social issues in nursing (Desantis & Lipson, 2007). In an effort to understand individual reaction to illness, the NLN Committee further included, in 1937, the individual's cultural background in the guide (Desantis & Lipson, 2007). The American Academy of Nursing Expert Panel on Culturally Competent Care (as cited by Desantis & Lipson, 2007) published a white paper in 1992 with guidelines for culturally competent care education of students. The American Nurses Association (ANA, 1991, 1995, 2003), American Association of Colleges of Nursing (AACN, 1998, 1999, 2008), and the NLN (2005, 2009a, 2009b) have been vocal in asserting their commitment to cultural diversity and promotion of cultural competence in nursing education.

Diverse groups continue to manifest disparities in health status and health care access despite the integration of cultural competence in nursing education (AACN, 2008; Sullivan Commission, 2004). McFarland and Leininger (2002, 2006) strongly advocated for explicit TCN education in both undergraduate and graduate levels. According to McFarland and Leininger (2002), there are four ways of integrating TCN content into the curricula: (1) integrating concepts and principles into existing curriculum; (2) integrating modules or units into a curriculum, (3) integrating series of organized courses in a curriculum, and (4) offering a major program or substantive track in TCN (pp. 534–535). Along the same advocacy, Giger et al. (2007) called for developing knowledge, skills, and competencies among health care workers; this should be initiated and incorporated in the educational curricula. It is also critical to look at cultural competence education and how the knowledge, skills, and competencies may prepare practitioners for licensure.

While graduates of entry level programs—diploma, associate, and baccalaureate—are expected to pass the National Council Licensing Examination-RN® (NCLEX-RN) after program completion, question items on cultural diversity and promotion of cultural competences have not been fully integrated in the examination (Paquaio, 2007), although Desantis and Lipson (2007) indicated that the California State Board of Nursing specifically mandates the inclusion of cultural diversity into the nursing curricula. The current blueprint of the NCLEX-RN (National Council of State Boards of Nursing [NCSBN], 2010) does not specifically indicate a cultural diversity area although the major category of the four client needs of safe effective care environment; health promotion and maintenance; psychosocial integrity; and physiologic integrity could all have implications when caring for culturally diverse clients. The concept of integration of cultural diversity and promotion of cultural competence, whether programmatic or for licensure purposes, deserves serious consideration in order to meet the outcome of preparing practitioners who are ready to care for culturally diverse populations. Indicating specific topics in cultural diversity in the licensing examination will be a strong incentive for nursing schools to cover this area in nursing curricula, most likely with a separate course dedicated to cultural diversity and promotion of cultural competence.

There is more focus on cultural competence in the master's program. Three schools are currently offering master's level preparation in cultural competence: Augsburg College, Minneapolis, MN, has a Master of Arts in Transcultural Nursing in the Community; Ball State University, Muncie, IN, offers modules and assessments leading to MS in Nursing; and the University of Washington, School of Nursing, Department of Psychosocial and Community Health in Seattle has Master in Nursing in Advanced Practice Community Health Systems program (TCNS, 2011a). Among schools that offer TCN courses in the master's program include Kean University, Union, NJ; Madonna University College of Nursing and Health in Livonia, MI; Medical University of Ohio College of Nursing in Toledo, OH; Mount Saint Mary College (MSMC) Division of Nursing, Newburgh, NY; Samford University Ida Moffett School of Nursing, Birmingham, AL; University of California at Los Angeles, CA (also open to doctoral students); University of North Dakota College of Nursing in Grand Forks, ND; and University of Saint Francis, Joliet, IL (TCNS, 2011a).

TCN Content: Integration of Concepts Versus Separate Courses

Despite advocates for formal teaching of TCN concepts in nursing curricula, there are no standardized guidelines for integration of content. Transcultural concepts are incorporated in nursing curricula but there is a wide variation in terms of "content, depth, and level of integration" (Ryan, Carlton, & Ali, 2000, p. 300). Although there is agreement that there is a need to prepare graduates who have the knowledge, skills, and attitudes to care for multicultural clients, families, groups, and communities, the means to achieve this common end vary in different schools.

In a national survey of baccalaureate and higher degree NLN-accredited schools, Ryan et al. (2000) found that only 89 undergraduate and 27 graduate schools had formal courses in TCN; the rest of the programs integrate TCN concepts in varying depth and breadth in the undergraduate program. Specifically, the Ryan et al. (2000) findings indicated that among undergraduate programs out of those surveyed, TCN courses are integrated into existing courses, 197 (214); modules in course, 135 (202); formal courses, 89 (205); and in the graduate programs, the figures were as follows: integrated into existing courses, 86 (115); modules, 56 (110), formal courses, 27 (103). Ryan et al. (2000) originally surveyed 610 schools but only had 36% survey return. Follow-up national surveys are needed and it is imperative to explore how baccalaureate programs prepare graduates with the knowledge, skills, and competencies to care for culturally diverse patients.

Another example of varying degrees of integration of transcultural concepts in nursing curricula is a Health Resources Services Administration (HRSA)-funded project at a university in the southern United States that implemented four modules across the master's program in nursing administration and leadership (Tuck, Moon, & Allocca, 2010). Tuck et al. (2010) chose Campinha-Bacote's Biblically Based Model of Cultural Competence in the Delivery of Healthcare Services (2005a, 2005b) mainly for the inclusion of cultural desire as a vital part of the model.

To explore teaching and learning methods involved incorporating cultural competence in the curricula, Lipson and Desantis (2007) conducted a survey of schools by telephone, electronic mail, and face–face interviews. Their findings indicate that knowledge, attitudes, and skills in cultural competence are included in nursing programs through (1) specialty focus, (2) required courses, (3) models, (4) immersion experiences, and (5) distance learning or simulation (Lipson & Desantis, 2007). Specialties at the MS level may comprise three or more courses in cultural competence in addition to other program requirements. In some schools, required nursing courses may vary: "transcultural nursing, cross-cultural nursing…health and culture, diversity…health disparities" (Lipson & Desantis, 2007, p. 12S). Lipson and Desantis concluded that some schools use the following theory and models, mainly those of Leininger, Purnell, Campinha-Bacote, Giger and Davidhizar, whereas other programs develop courses around books such as those of Andrews and Boyle and Spector—yet it is difficult to determine the actual number of schools and the models used.

The 1-year program to prepare licensed practical nurses, whether offered at a community college or in the last year of high school, is packed with courses in knowledge, skills, and competencies. Adding a separate course seems out of the question. However, it still is possible to integrate learning into existing assignments. For example, an assignment about Ellis and Liberty Islands could be used to spark empathy and compassion about diverse cultures and their means of immigration to this country. If a field trip is an impossibility, an Internet and other search are feasible; so is a short video about the migration from all over the world and how those people contributed to the making of the United States as a diverse, proud land.

Nursing schools still are mostly integrating TCN concepts in their curricula. The danger of curricular integration where there is no standardized content nor competencies is emphatically lamented by Boyle (2007): "…these courses are here today and gone tomorrow" (p. 21S). Nurse educators have diverse passions and may integrate aspects of those passions in the curricula—indeed when they leave—there is no guarantee that the integrated content will continue. We cannot afford such "hit or miss" teaching of TCN. Making way for required content in nursing curricula usually results in elimination of cultural content (Boyle, 2007).

The AACN (2008) adoption of models developed by Campinha-Bacote, Giger and Davidhizar, Leininger, Purnell, and Spector in its faculty toolkit for integration of cultural competence will probably show an increasing use of theory and models in education and later in practice and administration. One of the models used by the NLN in its *Commitment to Diversity in Nursing and Nursing Education* is Giger and Davidhizar's (2008) transcultural assessment model. In addition, continued mandates from accrediting bodies such as the Commission on Collegiate Nursing Education (CCNE) and National League for Nursing Accrediting Commission (NLNAC) and State Board of Nursing guidelines will continue to call for standardized content in nursing curricula or for separate course in cultural competence both in the undergraduate and graduate programs. Preparing graduates who have knowledge, skills, and attitudes to care for multicultural clients, families, groups, and communities or for licensure necessitate such standardization.

Furthermore, in the future more schools will elect to offer a separate course in TCN in both undergraduate and graduate curricula due to more and more outcome-based studies revealing the connection between disparities in care among minority populations and the number of minorities in the health care workforce. There is a renewed and continued commitment to increasing the number of ethnically diverse nurses in the health care workforce (AACN, 2008; NLN, 2005, 2009a, 2009b; Sullivan Commission, 2004).

Cultural Competence Among Nursing Students

Literature shows a gap in the area of research regarding the development of cultural competence among nursing students; this area is a fertile ground for further research in the future. The question also arose whether measuring cultural competence after graduation when nurses have been working would yield more meaningful results than measuring that competence when these nurses were students (Kardong-Edgreen & Campinha-Bacote, 2008; Lipson & Desantis, 2007).

In their study using the *Inventory for Assessing the Process of Cultural Competence* (IAPCC-R) among 212 U.S. baccalaureate students in four diverse programs, Kardong-Edgreen and Campinha-Bacote (2008) found out that the students only scored as culturally aware. Campinha-Bacote (2008) recognized the possibility of lack of reliability of the IAPCC-R and its limitation as a quantitative tool and further suggested using the student version of the IAPCC along with qualitative measures such as field notes and journaling.

Another study measured attitudinal and behavioral changes among baccalaureate students at a nursing program in the midwest using the Giger-Davidhizar model across the curriculum (Hughes & Hood, 2007). Subsequent measurement of student cross-cultural interaction with the Freeman's (1993, as cited in Hughes & Hood, 2007) Cross-Cultural Evaluation Tool (CCET) revealed consistent increase in scores among students in all levels of the curriculum. According to Hughes and Hood (2007), the CCET only measures attitudinal and behavioral changes; hence a tool that measures knowledge, skills, and competence may yield a more comprehensive result. Using a TCN model and determining its outcome from across courses and levels of the curriculum may be the best way to measure changes in students' cultural knowledge, skills, and competencies.

Lowe and Archibald (2009) emphatically called for increasing the diversity of nursing faculty. A culturally diverse faculty provide role models to students and help "interpret cultural knowledge and needs of diverse nursing students" (Lowe & Archibald, 2009, p. 15).

Faculty Preparation in TCN

There is increasing scrutiny of faculty preparation in TCN as we look at cultural competence among nursing students and the competence desired for practitioners ready to meet the health care needs of the growing number of culturally diverse population. Nursing faculty need formal preparation in TCN "...to ensure quality-based teaching and guidance as they need to shift from traditional nursing knowledge to largely new and unfamiliar knowledge in transcultural nursing" (Leininger, 2002c, p. 7). Over the years, evidence of faculty preparation in TCN has been disappointing. In 2002, McFarland and Leininger quoted that only 20% of faculty had formal education in TCN. Prior to becoming effective teachers, mentors, facilitators, and role models, faculty must first have formal education in the goals, scope, theories, practices, and outcomes of TCN (McFarland & Leininger, 2002) and must have passion about TCN (Lowe & Archibald, 2009). There is an urgent need for recruitment for graduate-prepared faculty in TCN not just for the United States but worldwide (McFarland & Leininger, 2002). This call to action from McFarland and Leininger, written in a chapter of their textbook *Transcultural Nursing: Concepts, Theories, Research, and Practice* in 2002, is as relevant then as it is now as we go further into the 21st century.

From a national survey of 610 NLN schools (217 responded), Ryan et al. (2000) cited 80 programs with faculty that have no preparation in TCN. The number of schools, along with the number of faculty with preparation in TCN for the rest of the schools surveyed, were as follows: 56 (1–2), 19 (3–4), 9 (5–8), 2 (13) (Ryan et al., 2000). While the result from the survey was promising, the researchers cautioned readers about the limitations of the study such as small sampling, linguistic variations of questions that may have led to higher number of responses, and wide variations in the interpretation of "preparation of faculty" whereby responses may be for exposure to other cultures by travel or international nursing experience rather than formal TCN preparation (Ryan et al., 2000).

Another study aimed at measuring faculty cultural competence was conducted by Sealy, Burnett, and Johnson (2006), a statewide survey among 313 (157 responded) baccalaureate program faculty in Louisiana. Sealy et al. (2006) administered the *Cultural Diversity Questionnaire for Nurse Educators*, an instrument developed by the researchers as well as items from Campinha-Bacote's (2003b, 2005a) model. The tool measures both an overall cultural competence score and provides a measure of each of these five components of culture: knowledge, skill, desire, encounter, and awareness (Sealy et al., 2006). The faculty in the Sealy et al. (2006) study scored highest in cultural awareness (4.14) but lowest in the subscale for cultural encounter (3.56), an evidence of the need to more encounters with clients of diverse cultures. While the overall score for cultural competence was 3.73 out of scale of 5, Sealy et al. (2006) indicated that this appears to "fall short" (p. 139) of the level expected for those responsible for preparing culturally competent nurses. Consequently, faculty are encouraged to attend continuing education programs in cultural competence to enhance their preparation in this area (Sealy et al., 2006). Similarly, among senior baccalaureate students, in a study that also used Campinha-Bacote's IAPCC-R scored highest in the awareness level (Kardong-Edgreen & Campinha-Bacote, 2008). How are we doing indeed after more than 25 years since the ANA first issued its guidelines in cultural diversity? Follow-up research in the area of faculty preparation in cultural competence needs to be a priority for current and future research.

The ANA (1991, 1995, 2003) has been consistent in its position about cultural diversity and the inclusion of culturally congruent care in all nurse–patient interactions. AACN (1998, 1999, 2008) and the NLN (and their accrediting bodies, CCNE and NLNAC, respectively) have continued to include cultural diversity and promotion of cultural competence as a top priority in nursing curricula. This and the increasing mandates, availability of resources, and research from The Joint Commission (2005, 2010a, 2010b) about linguistic and cultural competence in clinical practice have gained the impetus to critically appraise curricular content (Leininger, 2002c; McFarland & Leininger, 2002; Lipson & Desantis, 2007; Ryan et al., 2000); cultural competence of faculty, students, and graduates (Hughes & Hood, 2007; Kardong-Edgreen & Campinha-Bacote, 2008; Sealy et al., 2006); and the vital connection between increasing diversity in nursing schools and reducing disparities in health and health care (AACN, 2010; Fink, 2009; Lowe & Archibald, 2009; Pacquaio, 2007; Sullivan Commission, 2004). Gaps in knowledge in this area need to be research priority (Kardong-Edgreen & Campinha-Bacote, 2008). Along this line, Anderson, Calvillo, and Fongwa (2007) highlighted the interconnected roles of community partnerships with culturally competent nursing education, clinical practice and research; these linkages could have a promising outcome of reducing health disparities among vulnerable populations. Through a concept analysis, Fink (2009) cited four interventions to address health disparities: (1) providing culturally competent care;

(2) facilitation of cross cultural communication; (3) adding minorities as staff and administrators into the health profession; and (4) engaging in culturally competent research.

Nontraditional and Minority Students

Almost everyone trying to complete a nursing degree complains about the rigor of the program. The difficulty could be magnified by being a minority student and a nontraditional student. Some models are available for recruitment, engagement, retention, and success of minority and nontraditional students (Gilchrist & Rector, 2007; Jeffreys, 2004, 2012 [in press]; McFarland, Mixer, Lewis, & Easley, 2006). Furthermore, Pacquaio (2007) linked two important topics: cultural competence education and increasing the diversity in schools of nursing and in clinical practice settings to reduce the disparities in health care.

Nursing students from diverse cultures need understanding and caring (Leininger, 1995a), and the CCDU has shown its applicability in the recruitment, engagement, and retention of culturally diverse nursing students (McFarland et al., 2006) as they navigate academia in the journey to completion of the nursing program. Leininger (1995c, 2002c, 2006b) had long been an advocate for the inclusion of transcultural concepts in nursing curricula); the last years of this decade show the increased attention to this focus. The next decade, by many indications, will call for standardized content in the curricula as the primacy of cultural competence gains momentum and points to best evidence in narrowing the disparities in health care.

Gilchrist and Rector (2007) reviewed programatic initiatives such as HRSA's Kids Into Health Careers and formulated suggestions for best practices in education such as faculty development and student support. The faculty role is vital in the retention and success of nursing students. Faculty development must address (1) development of cultural knowledge, skills, competencies; (2) learning about the unique needs of culturally diverse nursing students; and (3) strategies to promore student recruitment, retention, and success (Gilchrist & Rector, 2007). Gilchrist and Rector suggested the following best practices for the recruitment, retention, and success of students: English as a Second Language training; faculty support in advising and mentoring; peer tutoring; and NCLEX preparation. Nursing's pursuit for culturally diverse workforce is attainable but the journey is just beginning (Gilchrist & Rector, 2007).

Jeffreys (2004) developed the *nursing undergraduate retention and success (NURS) model,* initally the nontraditonal undergraduate retention and success, to examine retention and success among nontraditional undergraduate nursing students. At the center of the NURS model are professional integration factors such as "nursing faculty advisement and helpfulness, memberships in professional organizations, professional events, encouragement by friends in class, enrichment programs, and peer mentoring and tutoring" (Jeffreys, 2004, p. 104). Integration factors are central because they represent the turning point of the decision by the student to persevere, drop out, or stop (Jeffreys, 2004). The faculty role is indeed vital in the retention of students. There are similarities in the support programs that Jeffreys(2004) and Gilchrist and Rector (2007) presented as retention strategies. Jeffreys (2004) book *Nursing Student Retention:Understanding the Process of Making A Difference* is now being revised for a second edition with a digital toolkit that will help educators ascertain reasons for loss of students and retention of students (Jeffreys, 2012 [in press]).

The Project Opportunities for Professional Education in Nursing (OPEN) received a 3-year federal grant to enable culturally diverse, educationally and/or finacially disadvantaged students enter and succeed in the baccalaureate program at a university in the midwest United States (McFarland et al., 2006). The project evaluators used Leininger's CCDU theory and Sunrise Enabler (1995a, 2002a) in all three phases of project OPEN: recruitment, engagement, and retention. According to McFarland et al. (2006), project services such as tutoring, prenursing coursework and advisement, writing support, financial aid, and cultural enrichment programs were adopted by the college of nursing and the university and preserved after the program. Leininger's CCDU theory and the sunrise enabler is an applicable framework that other schools of nursing could use to recruit, engage, and retain culturally diverse students.

Learning TCN at a Distance

Leininger pioneered distance delivery of TCN with the use of telelecture series within the United States and Oceania, Pacific Islands, as early as 1967 (McFarland & Leininger, 2002). Technology has advanced and many transcultural programs are delivered online in a synchronous (real time) or asynchronous (delayed time), transcending time and distance (O'Neil, Fisher, & Newbold, 2004). The online delivery is advantageous for nurses who live a distance from schools and for those who juggle personal, family, and professional responsibilities. Technology delivered courses are fully online and have no face-to-face meetings whereas hybrid or blended classes are combination of face-to-face and online (O'Neil et al., 2004), combining the best of both delivery modalities. Advances in communication and technology have created a world that has global interconnectedness and interdependencies (Andrews, 2006). Indeed, with a click of a mouse, it is possible to have dialogue with colleagues all over the world, to participate in webinars and conferencing, or to access the latest research and best practices from scholarly databases. These advances have enhanced the delivery of distance education in general and of TCN in particular.

Excelsior College's distance learning program has a long experience and hence has been able to develop and refine their program (Lipson & Desantis, 2007). Located in Albany, NY, Excelsior College School of Nursing is the world's largest educator of nurses at a distance; its baccalaureate program requires completion of a course regarding teaching and learning in a diverse society (Excelsior College, 2011). The College of Staten Island, City University of New York and Duquesne University in Pittsburgh, PA, both have online programs in Advanced Certificate in Cultural Competence (TCNS, 2011). MSMC in Newburgh, NY, requires a transcultural course in its master's programs and offers this in blended format (MSMC Bulletin, 2011). TCN concepts are integrated in all undergraduate nursing courses at MSMC.

Some critiques of distance programs include focus on provider–patient encounter and not paying attention to economic and political contexts affecting client's abilities to adhere to treatment. In cross-cultural courses, discussions could be enriched with having students from all over the world (Purnell, 2007). Having cultural care scenarios without any medical or nursing diagnoses enable students to work in groups as they analyze the scenario with the appropriate cultural domains along with the primary and secondary characteristics of culture (Purnell, 2007). Another way of networking efforts in TCN is through electronic collaboration; as an example, the "Community of Communities" at the School of Nursing at Ball State University where local, national, and international students and faculty may access the site and participate in dialogue and exchange about case studies and transcultural concepts (Ryan et al., 2000).

SECTION 3. NURSING PRACTICE

The National Sample Survey of Registered Nurses (NSSRN), initiated since 1977 and conducted every 4 years, provides the largest survey of registered nurses (RNs) in the United States. The data from NSSRN are vital in assessing (1) status in the United States nursing workforce; (2) responsiveness of workforce to federal and state programs that ensures enough nurses to provide essential health care services; (3) education and skills of nurses; (4) diversity of RNs and impact of foreign educated nurses; (5) factors affecting RN's decisions to engage in the nursing profession; and (6) future supply of RNs (U.S. Department of Health and Human Services [USDHHS], HRSA, 2010).

The largest group of health care workers in the United States are nurses. As of March 2008, an approximate 3,063,163 of RNs live in the United States; this number reflects an increase of 5.3% from 2004 or a growth of 153,806 RNs (USDHHS, HRSA, 2010). While there is a growth, the Labor Statistics project a need for more than a million new RNs by 2016 (as cited by AACN, 2010).

A comparison among initial nursing education of RNs between 2004 and 2008 showed a continued trend of increasing numbers of RNs prepared at the baccalaureate (from 31% to 33.7%), and associate (from 42.9% to 45.4%) degrees and a decrease in numbers of RNs with a diploma in nursing (from 25.6% to 20.4%) (USDHHS, HRSA, 2010). These trends have implications in nursing practice, education, and administration. Faculty members need to plan accordingly when integrating diversity and cultural competence in nursing curricula.

Missing Persons

It is widely accepted that the current ethnic diversity of nurses do not reflect the people they serve (Sullivan Commission, 2004; USDHHS, HRSA, 2010). The NSSRN reported that their 2008 survey showed that while 65.6% of the U.S. population are non-Hispanic White, there are 83.2% of white non-Hispanic RNs. Further, the NSSRN (USDHHS, HRSA, 2010) report highlighted the underrepresentation of the following, with corresponding percent of the U.S. population: Hispanic/Latino, 3.6% (15.4%), Black/African American, 5.4% (12.2%), and American Indian (AI)/Alaska Native, 0.3% (0.8%). There is slight overrepresentation of Asians at 5.8 for 4.5% of the population, possibly due to significant number of RNs from the Philippines and India

(USDHHS, HRSA, 2010). In its 2009 to 2010 enrollment and graduations report, the AACN (2010) confirmed that majority of graduates from nursing schools are White. Less than 9% of the total number of nurses are African Americans, Hispanic Americans, and AIs whereas these account for 25% of the U.S. population (Sullivan Commission, 2004). There is a marked lack of minority nurses who could inspire individuals to seek health care. The Sullivan Commisssion (2004) further reported that the low numbers of minority health care professionals are contributing to the continued racial and ethnic disparities in cancer and human immunodeficiency virus/acquired immune deficiency syndrome among African Americans, Hispanic Americans, and AIs. Despite nursing's intention to be culturally diverse, there is poor representation of ethnic minorities in the profession (Lowe & Archibald, 2009).

Midwives among African Americans date back to the 17th century with the slave trade. The legacy continues on today as African American midwives render quality care to African Americans, Native Americans, and other low-income families (Ellerby-Brown, Sims, & Schorn, 2008). The American College of Nurse Midwives in 2003 (as cited in Ellerby-Brown et al., 2008) highlighted the lack of minority in the field with statistics showing less than 4% African Americans, 1% Asian, and less than 1% Native American among current midwives.

It is interesting to note that some programs are in place not only to increase enrollment of AI/Alaska natives but also to assure their successful program completion and prepare them for leadership to alleviate the marked disparities in health care among Native Americans (Shelton, 2008). Considering that less than 10% of baccalaureate and graduate nursing faculty are nurses of color (Ellerby-Brown et al., 2008), nursing education does not have enough role models. Among Native Americans, there are only 14 doctorally prepared nurses (Williams, 2008). One of them, Dr. John Lowe from the Cherokee Nation who is also an associate professor at Florida Atlantic University, has been conducting research for over 20 years to find solutions to the Indian health disparities. Lowe's master's thesis on the social support to reduce substance abuse started his career in seeking culturally competent solutions for health disparities among his own people (Williams, 2008). There is evidence that most minority nurses go back to their own community to care for their own people (Katz, O'Neil, Strickland, & Doutrich, 2010; Pacquiao, 2007; Williams, 2008). Nurses serving their own communities may eliminate health care disparities (Fink, 2009).

The review of 55 studies by Saha and Shipman in 2006 (as cited in Katz et al., 2010) revealed that minority health professionals tend to practice in minority communities and that clients reported more satisfactory interpersonal care when racial and ethnic harmony exist. Katz et al. (2010) found that although the nine nurse participants in their study reported a sense of tremendous loss for leaving—they came to a breaking point wherein the stress made them pysically ill—and they had to quit their jobs. While limited in sample, Katz et al. (2010) provided a poignant picture of a tug of war between the nurses' commitment to serve their own people and the difficulty and consequent inability to navigate hierarchical organizational systems. Currently, there is a paucity of studies exploring the impact of hiring and retention of culturally diverse nurses working in their original communities (Katz et al., 2010). This area calls for more funded research if the United States is to reach its Healthy People objectives of increasing U.S. minority nurses (USDHHS, 2000).

Certification in TCN

The need for TCN certification was evident in the 1970s, as nurses struggled to care for immigrants, refugees, and other culturally diverse peoples (McFarland & Leininger, 2002). TCNS began its work in certification (CTN) in 1987 and administered the first examination in 1988 (McFarland & Leininger, 2002; TCNS, 2011). Purposes of certification include

- To provide quality-based and research-based cultural care knowledge for competent care practices;
- To recognize the expertise of transcultural nurses prepared to care for clients of diverse and similar cultures; and
- To maintain quality-based standards and policies for transcultural nursing practices (McFarland & Leininger, 2002, p. 544)

The written exam, composed of mostly multiple choice items, also included an oral examination and was usually given at the annual international TCNS conference. The CTN is prepared at the graduate level and usually assumes roles such as facilitating organizational competence; ensuring language access services; assisting patients and families in culturally based care; collaboration with the health care team for culturally competent care; and community outreach to develop health promotion programs (Curren, 2006).

In 2004, the TCNS Board of Trustees appointed a Certification Task Force to review current certification practices and to make recommendations in order to move the CTN certification on par with other current certification examinations. Upon the recommendation of the Task Force, the TCNS Board of Trustees established the Transcultural Nursing Certification Commission (TNCC) in 2006 (TCNS, 2011). The TCNCC worked extensively in creating updated guidelines for certification including two levels of certification: advanced (CTN-A) for those with master's degrees or higher, and a basic certification for diploma, associate, and baccalaureate-prepared nurses (CTN-B). Furthermore, the new certification examination deleted the verbal component in keeping with other specialty certification process. The new examination for advanced certification was given as pilot in January and February 2009; the second pilot exam was given in June and July 2009 (TCNS, 2010). Currently, a task force is in the process of developing the basic certification examination for implementation in 2011. The examination is available on Blackboard and is administered at strategic testing centers located all over the United States. Advanced and basic certification in TCN demonstrates that the nurse is an expert and qualified to guide colleagues, patients, and others in culturally competent care (Curren, 2006; TCNS, 2011). There are about 85 CTNs worldwide (P. Sagar, personal communication, March 10, 2011).

SECTION 4. NURSING ADMINISTRATION

The journey to cultural competence by individuals and organizations need supportive climate (Giger et al., 2007) and mentoring (Purnell, 2008). The journey is seen as a process, not end point (Andrews, 2008b; Campinha-Bacote, 2003a, 2005a, 2007; Galanti, 2008). Giger et al. (2007) also called for advocacy and policy making by the American Academy of Nursing along with research focused on disparities, diversity, and cultural competence to eliminate disparities in health care.

The diversity of the health care workforce has markedly increased over the years. This increased diversity calls for TCN administration (Andrews, 2008c). This type of administration requires leaders to examine the workforce's perspectives about work; values in the workplace; and cultural assessment of individuals as well as cultural assessment of the organization (Andrews, 2008a). Leininger's CCDU will be applicable in diverse organizational settings (Andrews & Boyle, 2008; Hubbert, 2006; Leininger, 1995b, 2002c, 2006b; Ludwig-Beymer, 2008).

Nurse Graduates of Foreign Nursing Schools

The numbers of nurse graduates of foreign nursing programs currently practicing in the United States as RNs have increased from 3.7% in 2004 to 5.6% in 2008 (USDHHS, HRSA, 2010). This increase is consistent with the growth of foreign educated nurses who passed the NCLEX in 2007 (22,000 nurses) compared to 1998 (5,000 nurses). Other developed countries such as the United Kingdom (Cowan & Norman, 2006) and Australia (Brunero et al., 2008) have also resorted to recruitment of foreign educated nurses.

Nurses immigrating from other countries face challenges as they undergo the process of acculturation and work professionally in the host country (Brunero et al., 2008; Cowan & Norman, 2006; DiCicco-Bloom, 2004; Pacquaio, 2007). In a study of 10 nurses born in Kerala, India, DiCicco-Bloom (2004) found three themes from the semi-structured interviews: cultural displacement; experience of racism and alienation; and intersections of categories of being a female nurse, an immigrant, and non-White. The nurses described cultural displacement as "a foot here, a foot there, a foot nowhere" (DiCicco-Bloom, 2004, p. 28). The nurses described a common feeling about immigrants when reconciling own traditions and culture with those of the new country and of feelings of being in two places at the same time. The conflict of the women were echoed by DiCicco-Bloom (2004) as the nurses clung to the past while staking a position in the present. The nurses narrated instances of disrimination and racism in the nursing profession, which is reflective of general society (DiCicco-Bloom, 2004). Consequently, DiCicco-Bloom urged nurses to be advocates against racism and discrimination in health care; she also suggested more research about experiences of foreign educated nurses as health care providers and as residents of the United States.

Ea, Griffin, L'Eplattenier, and Fitzpatrick (2008) conducted surveys among a convenient sample of 96 Filipino RNs at a Philippine Nurses Association of America (PNAA) convention. In this descriptive correlational study, the researchers administered the 12-item Short Acculturation Scale for Filipino Americans (de la Cruz et al., 2000) and Part B of the Index of Work Satisfaction. Results indicated a moderate level of job satisfaction, which correlated to a level of acculturation nearer American than Filipino culture (Ea et al., 2008). In addition, according to Ea et al. (2008), the nurse's age, length of stay (average = 15 years) in the United States, and acculturation are significant predictors of their perception of job satisfaction. The majority of Filipino nurses in this study were members of the PNAA, indicative of professional involvement in itself.

Brunero et al. (2008) discovered three themes in their study of 150 (56 returned the survey) foreign educated nurses in Sidney, Australia: career and lifestyle opportunities; differences in practice; and homesickness. Of the 56 nurses, 27 were from England; the rest of the nurses hailed from Canada (6), Ireland (3), Sweden (3), Fiji (1), Finland (2), the United States (2), Zimbabwe (2), China (1), New Zealand (1), Philippines (1), Singapore (1) (Brunero et al., 2008). Though the Brunero et al.(2008) sample is small, it revealed worldwide mobility of nurses. Cultural competence training for foreign educated nurses is necessary if they were to make the essential professional transition and acculturation in the new country. Quantifying the effects of cultural competence training among foreign educated nurses to their acculturation, professional adjustment, and personal satisfaction is a research priority and may identify knowledge gaps in terms of recruitment, engagement, and retention.

Pacquiao (2007) performed a 3-year outcome evaluation of an acculturation program for recruited nurses from India, the Philippines, and Trinidad and Tobago and for their managers, preceptors, and educators. The program consisted of verbal and written communication, leadership training, clinical judgment, and professional roles. The result of the 5-day intervention for the nurses and 2-day sessions for the managers, preceptors, and educators revealed positive outcomes: (1) increased empathy for patients and coworkers, (2) easier transition to organizational culture, and (3) improved teamwork and organizational support for diverse workforce development (Pacquaio, 2007). Mentoring programs for foreign educated nurses have also been suggested (International Council of Nurses, 2007; Purnell, 2008).

SECTION 5. FUTURE OF TRANSCULTURAL NURSING

It is an exciting time for TCN indeed. The germinal work of Dr. Leininger is closer to full fruition; much of her vision about TCN, succinctly implied in this statement: "that the culture needs of people in the world be met by nurses prepared in transcultural nursing" (Leininger, 1995b), is at the crossroads. As the United States becomes more diverse, there is a challenge that we need to confront whether we are in academia, in the practice arena, or in administration. Leininger, just like Florence Nightingale, was way ahead of her time. Leininger's blending of two worlds of nursing and anthropology brings one in awe of her persistence and inspiring work to lay the ground work for TCN.

Leininger's (1995a, 2006a) ethnonursing method has frequently been used as conceptual framework in qualitative research. Leininger's work—and those who follow—had created, is creating, and will further create body of evidence-based knowledge in TCN. Admittedly, more research is needed especially in areas of disparity in health care. This body of knowledge will be used in nursing education, practice, and administration well into the 21st century and will further narrow the gaps that exist in health care among marginalized groups and vulnerable populations versus those of the mainstream population.

Although nursing schools still are mostly integrating TCN concepts in their curricula, in the future more schools will likely elect to offer separate courses in TCN in both undergraduate and graduate curricula. Among undergraduate nursing curricula, overcrowding is one reason many schools find it difficult to add a separate course in cultural diversity and promotion of cultural competence. How can we not afford a three-credit class in TCN when we can afford eight credits in chemistry? Have we embraced holism in theory but in practice care for the body separately from the mind and the spirit? How can we get away from the medical model and truly practice holistic culturally congruent care? More and more outcome-based studies are emerging revealing the connection between disparities in care among minority populations and the number of culturally diverse workers (Sullivan Commission, 2004). There is a renewed and continued commitment to increasing the number of ethnically diverse nurses in the health care workforce (AACN, 2008; NLN, 2005, 2009a, 2009b; Sullivan Commission, 2004).

Call to Action To All Nurses: From Cultural Broker to Cultural Activist

Numbering approximately 3,063,163 according to the U.S. NSSRN, nurses are the largest group of professional health care workers (USDHHS, HRSA, 2010). There is strength in number; a potential that nurses have not totally capitalized on. If nurses heed the call for cultural knowledge, skills, and competencies in TCN and apply these in whatever settings they are engaged in—caring for clients in the home, in communities, and in institutions; teaching and preparing the next generation of nurses; or in leading academia and organizations—the outcomes will be truly significant. There and then, maybe nurses could truly make a difference in narrowing the diparities in access, provision, and quality of care among vulnerable and minority populations.

These vulnerable people, already disadvantaged, will not feel like they are grabbing at a double-edged sword each time they access and use health care resources.

The ground meat parable is indeed a "telling commentary of the urgent need for culturally competent care delivery in our diverse world" (Ford, 2009, p. 99). In this parable, Ford (2009) narrated how a refugee eloquently explained why refugees will not verbalize the pains of grabbing at a double-edged sword as salvation measure while drowning in the river of needs. It is a poignant description, an allegory of substandard care and quality for vulnerable populations. The verbalization came out as helpers asked the refugees for correction if they become insensitive to those being helped. Ford also pointed out that the young undergraduate students did not understand the refugee's story—a proof that, indeed, we all need to facilitate effective communication.

Gray and Thomas (2005) posed thought-provoking challenges for nursing as we continue to be mindful of inclusion of culture and cultural competence in nursing education, urging nursing education to move beyond cultural brokering to cultural activism. Concerned that the current nursing literature promotes that of a capitalistic, ethnocentric culture, it is imperative that we look at the rich heritage of social activism entrenched in nursing's beginning—from that of Nightingale's involvement in Scutari, Wald's work in establishing the Henry Street Settlement in New York, Dock's effort in fighting for suffrage, and Breckenridge's toil in establishing the Frontier Nursing Service (Gray & Thomas, 2005; Stanhope & Lancaster, 2010). It is right and fitting to include Leininger among these great nurses (Ryan, 2010). We also need to acknowledge the emerging leaders of TCN who have enriched the field with their own contributions: Andrews, Boyle, Campinha-Bacote, Davidhizar, Giger, McFarland, Purnell, and Spector, to name just a few. We all could have our own visions of what TCN could be—a force directing our teaching, our practice, our leading, and our research.

The readers and users of this book are encouraged to go back to the original theory, models, and guide as they try to select one that "fits" or is congruent with the mission, philosophy, and goals of each of their own settings. In addition, it is imperative to also see the fit between current mandates and guidelines with the components of each theory, models, and guide. The challenge, according to Douglas (2002), is to test your choice of theory, model, or guide as you apply it in education, practice, and administration and to identify gaps in knowledge for further research. It is only then that the theory, models, and guide are allowed to be what they are meant to be: growing, evolving, and being tested in order to survive (Douglas, 2002). In the process, they add to the body of knowledge in evidence-based practice (EBP) and show gaps for further research; guide clinical practice and organizations; and direct education and preparation of future practitioners in health care. The need and the urgency are upon us. The time is now.

REFERENCES

American Nurses Association. (1991). *Position statement on cultural diversity in nursing practice.* Kansas City, MO: Author.

American Nurses Association. (1995). *Nursing's social policy statement.* Washington, DC: Author.

American Nurses Association. (2003). *Nursing's social policy statement* (2nd ed.). Washington, DC: Nurses Books.

American Association of Colleges of Nursing. (1998). *The essentials of baccalaureate education for professional nursing practice.* Washington, DC: Author.

American Association of Colleges of Nursing. (1999). *Nursing education's agenda for the 21st century.* Washington, DC: Author

American Association of Colleges of Nursing. (2008). *Cultural competency in baccalaureate nursing education.* Washington, DC: Author.

Anderson, N. L. R., Calvillo, E. R., & Fongwa, M. N. (2007). Community-based approaches to strengthen cultural competency in nursing education and practice. *Journal of Transcultural Nursing, 18*(1), 49S–59S.

Andrews, M. M. (2006). The globalization of transcultural nursing theory and research. In M. M. Leininger & M. R. McFarland (eds.), *Culture care diversity and universality: A worldwide nursing theory* (2nd ed., pp. 83–114). Sudbury, MA: Jones & Bartlett.

Andrews, M. M. (2008a). Cultural competence in the health history and physical examination. In M. M. Andrews & J. S. Boyle (Eds.), *Transcultural concepts in nursing care* (5th ed., pp. 34–65). Philadelphia, PA: Wolters Kluwer/Lippincott Williams & Wilkins.

Andrews, M. M. (2008b). Culturally competent nursing care. In M. M Andrews & J. S. Boyle (Eds.), *Transcultural concepts in nursing care* (5th ed., pp. 15–33). Philadelphia, PA: Wolters Kluwer/Lippincott Williams & Wilkins.

Andrews, M. M. (2008c). Cultural diversity in the health care workforce. In M. M. Andrews & J. S. Boyle (Eds.), *Transcultural concepts in nursing care* (5th ed., pp. 297–326). Philadelphia, PA: Wolters Kluwer/Lippincott Williams & Wilkins.

Berry-Caban, C. S., & Crespo, H. (2008). Cultural competency as a skill for health care providers. *Hispanic Health International, 6*(3), 115–121.

Boyle, J. S. (2007). Commentary on "current approaches to integrating elements of cultural competence in nursing education." *Journal of Transcultural Nursing, 18*(1), 21S–22S.

Campinha-Bacote, J. (2003b). Many faces: Addressing diversity in health care. *Journal of Issues in Nursing, 8*(1), 16–22. Retrieved November 16,

2010, from http://www.nursingworld.org/MainMenuCategories/ANA Marketplace/ANAPeriodicals/OJIN/TableofContents/Volume82003/No1Jan2003/AdressingDiversityinHealthCare.aspx

Campinha-Bacote, J. (2005a). *A Biblically based model of cultural competence in the delivery of healthcare services.* Cincinnati, OH: Transcultural C.A.R.E. Associates.

Campinha-Bacote, J. (2005b). A Biblically based model of cultural competence in healthcare delivery. *Journal of Multicultural Nursing & Health, 11*(2), 16–22.

Campinha-Bacote, J. (2008). Cultural desire: 'Caught' or 'taught'? *Contemporary Nurse, 28,* 141–148.

Cowan, D. T., & Norman, I (2006). Cultural competence in nursing: New meanings. *Journal of Transcultural Nursing, 17*(1), 82–88.

Curren, D. A. (2006). Culture care needs in the clinical setting. In M. M. Leininger & M. R. McFarland (Eds.), *Transcultural nursing: Concepts, theories, research, and practice* (3rd ed., pp. 159–180). New York, NY: McGraw-Hill.

Desantis, L. A., & Lipson, J. G. (2007). Brief history of inclusion of content on culture in nursing education. *Journal of Transcultural Nursing, 18*(1), 7S–9S.

DiCicco-Bloom, B. (2004). The racial and gendered expereinces of immigrant nurses from Kerala, India. *Journal of Transcultural Nursing, 15*(1), 26–33.

Dobbins, M., Ciliska, D., Estabrooks, C., & Hayward. (2005). Changing nursing practice in an organization. In A. DiCenso, G. Guyatt, & D. Ciliska (Eds.), *Evidence-based nursing: A guide to clinical practice* (pp. 172–200). St. Louis, MO: Elsevier Mosby.

Douglas, M. (2002). Developing frameworks for providing culturally competent health care (Editorial). *Journal of Transcultural Nursing, 13*(3), 177.

Ea, E. E., Griffin, M., L'Eplattenier, N., & Fitzpatrick, J. J. (2008). Job satisfaction and acculturation among Filipino registered nurses. *Journal of Nursing Scholarship, 40*(1), 46–51.

Ellerby-Brown, A., Sims, T., & Schorn, M. (2008). African American nurse-midwives: Continuing the legacy. *Minority Nurse, 46–49.*

Excelsior College. (2011). *School of nursing.* Albany, NY: Author. Retrieved February 19, 2011, from http://www.excelsior.edu/school-of-nursing

Fink, A. M. (2009). Toward a new definition of health disparity. *Journal of Transcultural Nursing, 20*(4), 349–357.

Ford, V. (2009). Nursing perspectives in addressing health disparities. In S. Kosoko-Lasaki, C. T. Cook, & R. L. O'Brien (Eds.), *Cultural proficiency in addressing health disparities* (pp. 87–101). Sudbury, MA: Jones & Bartlett.

Galanti, G. A. (2008). *Caring for patients from different cultures.* Philadelphia, PA: University of Pennsylvania Press.

Giger, J. N., Davidhizar, R. E., Purnell, L., Harden, J. T., Phillips, J., & Strickland, O. (2007). American Academy of Nursing expert panel report: Developing cultural comptence to eliminate health disparities in ethnic minorities and other vulnerable populations. *Journal of Transcultural Nursing, 18*(2), 95–102.

Gilchrist, K. L., & Rector, C. (2007). Can you keep them? Strategies to attract and retain nursing students from diverse populations: Best practices in nursing education. *Journal of Transcultural Nursing, 18*(3), 277–285.

Glittenberg, J. (2004). A transdisciplinary, transcultural model for health care. *Journal of Transcultural Nursing, 15*(1), 6–10.

Gray, P., & Thomas, D. (2005). Critical analysis of "culture" in nursing literature: Implications for nursing education in the United States. In M. H. Oermann (Ed) and K. T. Heinrich (Associate Ed.), *Annual review of nursing education: Strategies for teaching, assessment, and program planning* (pp. 249–270). New York, NY: Springer.

Hughes, K. H., & Hood, L. J. (2007). Teaching methods and an outcome tool for measuring cultural sensitivity in undergraduate nursing students. *Journal of Transcultural Nursing, 18*(1), 57–62.

Hubbert, A. (2006). Application of culture care theory for clinical nurse administrators and managers. In M. Leininger & M. McFarland (Eds.), *Culture care diversity and universality: A worldwide nursing theory* (pp. 349–364). Boston, MA: Jones & Bartlett.

International Council of Nurses. (2007). Ethical nurse recruitment position paper. Retrieved September 17, 2009, from http://www.icn.ch/psrecruit01.htm#ftn1

Jeffreys, M. R. (2004). *Nursing student retention: Understanding the process and making a difference.* New York, NY: Springer.

Jeffreys, M. R. (in Press, 2012). *Nursing student retention: Understanding the process and making a difference* (2nd ed.). New York, NY: Springer.

Kardong-Edgreen, S., & Campinha-Bacote, J. (2008). Cultural competency of graduating US Bachelor of science nursing students. *Contemporary Nurse, 28,* 37–44.

Katz, J. R., O'Neil, G., Strickland, C. J., & Doutrich, D. (2010). Retention of Native American nurses working in their communities. *Journal of Transcultural Nursing, 21*(4), 393–401.

Leininger, M. M. (1995b). Types of health practitioners and cultural imposition. In M. Leininger (Ed.), *Transcultural nursing: Concepts, theories, research, and practice* (2nd ed., pp. 173–186). New York, NY: McGraw-Hill Companies.

Leininger, M. M. (1995c). Teaching transcultural nursing in undergraduate and graduate nursing programs. In M. Leininger (Ed.), *Transcultural nursing: Concepts, theories, research, and practice* (2nd ed., pp. 605–625). New York, NY: McGraw-Hill Companies.

Leininger, M. M. (2002a). Culture care theory: A major contribution to advance transcultural nursing knowledge and practices. *Journal of Transcultural Nursing, 13*(3), 189–192.

Leininger, M. M. (2002c). Transcultural nursing administration and consultation. In M. Leininger & M. McFarland (Eds.), *Transcultural nursing: Concepts, theories, research, and practice* (3rd ed., pp. 563–573). New York, NY: McGraw-Hill Companies.

Leininger, M. M. (2006a). Culture care diversity and universality and evolution of the ethnonursing method. In M. Leininger & M. McFarland (Eds.), *Culture care diversity and universality: A worldwide nursing theory* (pp. 1–41). Boston, MA: Jones & Bartlett.

Leininger, M. M. (2006b). Culture care theory and uses in nursing administration. In M. Leininger & M. McFarland (Eds.), *Culture care diversity and universality: A worldwide nursing theory* (pp. 365– 379). Boston, MA: Jones & Bartlett.

Leininger, M. M., & McFarland, M. (2006). *Culture care diversity and universality: A worldwide nursing theory.* Boston, MA: Jones & Bartlett.

Lipson, J. G., & Desantis, L. A. (2007). Current approaches to integrating elements of cultural competence in nursing education. *Journal of Transcultural Nursing, 18*(1), 10S–20S.

Lowe, J., & Archibald, C. (2009). Cultural diversity: The intention of nursing. *Nursing Forum, 44*(1), 11–18.

Ludwig-Beymer, P. (2008). Creating culturally competent organizations. In M. M. Andrews & J. S. Boyle (Eds.), *Transcultural concepts in nursing* (5th ed.). Philadelphia, PA: Wolters Kluwer Health/Lippincott, Williams, & Wilkins.

McFarland, M. R., & Leininger, M. M. (2002). Transcultural nursing: Curricular concepts, principles, and teaching and learning activities for the 21st century. In M. M. Leininger & M. R. McFarland (Eds.), *Transcultural nursing: Concepts, theories, research, and practice* (3rd ed., pp. 527–561). New York, NY: McGraw-Hill.

McFarland, M., Mixer, S., Lewis, A. E., & Easley, C. (2006). Use of the culture care theory as a framework for the recruitment, engagement,and retention of culturally diverse nursing students in a traditionally European American baccalaureate nursing program. In M. Leininger and M. McFarland (Eds.), *Culture care diversity and universality: A worldwide nursing theory* (pp. 239–254). Boston, MA: Jones & Bartlett.

National Council of State Boards of Nursing. (2010). *NCLEX-RN test plan.* Chicago, IL: Author. Retrieved February 10, 2010, from https://www.ncsbn.org/2010_NCLEX_RN_TestPlan.pdf

O'Neil, C. A., Fisher, C. A., & Newbold, S. K. (2004). *Developing an online course: Best practices for nurse educators.* New York, NY: Springer.

Mount Saint Mary College. (2011). *Graduate catalog: Master of science of nursing.* Newburgh, NY: Author.

National League for Nursing. (2005). *Core competencies of nurse educators with task statements.* New York, NY: Author. Retrieved January 26, 2011, from NLN website: http://www.nln.org/aboutnln/core_competencies/cce_dial3.htm

National League for Nursing. (2009a). *A commitment ot diversity in nursing and nursing education.* Retrieved January 26, 2011, from NLN website: http://www.nln.org/aboutnln/reflection_dialogue/rfl_dial3.htm

National League for Nursing. (2009b). *Diversity toolkit.* Retrieved January 26, 2011, from NLN website: http://www.nln.org/aboutnln/reflection_dialogue/rfl_dial3.htm

Paquiao, D. (2007). The relationship between cultural competence education and increasing diversity in nursing schools and practice settings. *Journal of Transcultural Nursing, 18*(1), 28S–37S.

Purnell, L. D. (2007). Commentary on "current approaches to integrating elements of cultural competence in nursing education." *Journal of Transcultural Nursing, 18*(1), 25S–27S.

Ryan, M., Carlton, K. H., & Ali, N. (2000). Transcultural nursing concepts and experiences in nursing curricula. *Journal of Transcultural Nursing, 11*(4), 300–307.

Ryan, M. (2011). A celebration of a life of commitment to transcultural nursing: Opening of the Madeleine M. Leininger Collection on Human Caring and Transcultural Nursing. *Journal of Transcultural Nursing, 22*(1), 97.

Sealy, L. J., Burnett, M., & Johnson, G. (2006). Cultural competence of baccalaureate nursing faculty: Are we up to the task? *Journal of Cultural Diversity, 13*(3), 131–140.

Shelton, T. (2008). Putting Native American nursing students on the path to success. *Minority Nurse*, 52–56.

Stanhope, M., & Lancaster, J. (2010*). Foundations of nursing in the community: Community-oriented practice* (3rd ed.). St. Louis, MO: Mosby/Elsevier.

Sullivan Commission. (2004). Missing persons: Minorities in the health professions: A report of the Sullivan Commission on diversity in the health care workforce. Retrieved January 26, 2011, from www.jointcenter.org/healthpolicy/docs/Sullivan.pdf

The Joint Commission. (2010a). *Advancing effective communication, cultural competence, and patient- and family-centered care: A roadmap for hospitals.* Oakbrook Terrace, IL: Author.

The Joint Commission. (2010b). *Cultural and linguistic care in area hospitals.* Oakbrook Terrace, IL: Author.

Transcultural Nursing Society. (2011a). Programs of study leading to a master's degree or certification in transcultural nursing in the United States. Retrieved on February 19, 2011, from http://www.tcns.org/TCNCourses.html

Transcultural Nursing Society. (2011b). Transcultural nursing certification. Retrieved February 19, 2011, from http://www.tcns.org/Certification.html

Tuck, I., Moon, M. W., Allocca, P. N. (2010). An integrative approach to cultural comptence education for advanced practice nurses. *Journal of Transcultural Nursing, 21*(4), 402–409.

U.S. Department of Health and Human Services, Office of Minority Health. (2000). Culturally and linguistically appropriate services. Retrieved August 26, 2010, from http://www.usdhhs.gov

U.S. Department of Health and Human Services, Health Resources Services Administration. (2010). The Registered Nurse population: Initial findings from the 2008 National Sample Survey of registered nurses. Retrieved January 18, 2011, from bhpr.hrsa.gov/healthworkforce/rnsurveys/rnsurveyinitial2008.pdf - 2011-05-06

Williams, S. (2008). Lessons from my father. *Minority Nurse*, 40–44.

Answers

ANSWERS TO NCLEX-TYPE QUESTIONS

Chapter 1. Madeleine Leininger's Theory of Culture Care Diversity and Universality

1. B
2. C
3. B
4. A
5. B
6. D
7. C
8. A
9. D
10. C
11. A
12. C
13. B
14. A
15. C

Chapter 2. Larry Purnell's Model for Cultural Competence

1. A
2. A
3. B
4. D
5. C
6. B
7. A
8. C
9. C
10. A
11. D
12. B
13. B
14. A
15. D

Chapter 3. Josepha Campinha-Bacote's *The Process of Cultural Competence in the Delivery of Healthcare Services* and *Biblically Based Model of Cultural Competence*

1. A
2. D
3. D
4. D
5. B
6. C
7. A
8. A
9. B
10. C
11. B
12. D
13. C
14. C
15. D

Chapter 4. Joyce Newman Giger and Ruth Davidhizar's Transcultural Assessment Model

1. D
2. C
3. C
4. A
5. A
6. B
7. B
8. D
9. C
10. B
11. B
12. C
13. B
14. B
15. A

Chapter 5. Rachel Spector's Health Traditions Model

1. B
2. A
3. C
4. A
5. D
6. B
7. A
8. D
9. C
10. B
11. D
12. B
13. A
14. B
15. C

Chapter 6. Margaret Andrews/Joyceen Boyle
Transcultural Nursing Assessment Guide for
Individuals and Families

1. A
2. B
3. D
4. C
5. B
6. B
7. C
8. A
9. B
10. D
11. A
12. A
13. C
14. A
15. B
16. A

Appendix A

NEW YORK STATE NURSES ASSOCIATION

Educational Activity Overview

Lesson Plan. Using Leininger's Sunrise Model and Components Across Models.

Purpose: This program is offered to promote cultural competence among healthcare workers. Attendees will use information in the care of their multicultural clients and in dealing with culturally diverse coworkers.

Objectives	Content (Topics)	Time Frame	Presenter	Teaching Methods
Learner oriented with one measurable behavioral verb per objective.	Outline of the content to be covered that will enable the learners to meet their objectives.	State the time frame for each objective.	List the faculty or content expert for each objective.	Describe the teaching methods, strategies, materials, and resources for each objective.

(Continued)

Continued

Objectives	Content (Topics)	Time Frame	Presenter	Teaching Methods
At the completion of this workshop, the learner will:	Pretest	5 minutes	Dr. P. Sagar	Pretest PowerPoint presentation Question and answer AVs

1. Identify challenges and opportunities of a growing multicultural population and workforce.	I. Cultural diversity in the healthcare workforce
	a. Cultural perspectives on the meaning of work
	  i. Individualism
	  ii. Collectivism
		20 minutes		Discussion Case studies/ scenarios

	II. Cultural diversity among our patients, their families/ significant others a. Cultural competence: A Process			
	III. History of transcultural nursing a. Transcultural nursing society b. Journal of TCNS c. Challenges ahead			
	IV. Cultural assessment guide a. Individual b. Organizational			

(*Continued*)

Objectives	Content (Topics)	Time Frame	Presenter	Teaching Methods
2. Use Leininger's action strategies in the care of multicultural clients.	II. Leininger's Sunrise Model Three action strategies a. Preservation/ maintenance b. Accommodation/ negotiation c. Repatterning/ restructuring Application of model to care of African Americans Some research Filipino Americans Some research Mexican Americans Some research Italian Americans Some research Arab Americans Some research	20 minutes	Dr. P. Sagar	Case studies/ scenarios Nursing care plan Role playing PowerPoint presentation Case studies/ scenarios: African- Americans Mexican Americans AVs
3. Apply cultural standards guiding equitable care.	III. Guidelines: Cultural standards a. Nursing practice i. ANA ii. Office of Minority Health iii. CLAS standards iv. JCAHO standards v. Magnet criteria b. Critique: Are we in compliance with these standards?	15 minutes		Role playing Clinical examples Question and answer AVs

(Continued)

Continued

Objectives	Content (Topics)	Time Frame	Presenter	Teaching Methods

4. Identify barriers and facilitators when promoting harmony in the multicultural workforce.
 	
5. Enumerate culturally competent approaches in dealing with coworkers, patients, families and/or significant others.
	IV. Cultural Competence: Dealing with coworkers, patients, families, and/or significant others
	a. Cross-cultural communication
	  i. Touch
	  ii. Etiquette
	b. Clothing and accessories
	c. Time orientation
	d. Interpersonal relationships
	e. Gender and sexual orientation
	f. Moral and religious beliefs
	g. Creating a culturally competent organization: An ongoing process
	h. Promoting harmony in the multicultural workforce
	  i. Barriers
	  ii. Facilitators
	
	Follow up activities
	
	Ongoing approaches to cultural competence
	
	Evaluation and post test
		25 minutes
		
		5 minutes
			Dr. P. Sagar	Case studies/ scenarios
				Role playing
				PowerPoint presentation
				Question and answer
				Posttest
				Evaluation

Appendix B

NEW YORK STATE NURSES ASSOCIATION

Journey Into Cultural Competence

Lesson Plan. Using Campinha-Bacote's Model.
JOURNEY INTO CULTURAL COMPETENCE

Purpose: The program is offered to promote cultural competence among health care workers. Attendees will use information in the care of their multicultural clients.

Objectives	Content (Topics)	Time Frame	Presenter	Methods
List learner's objectives in behavioral terms	Provide an outline of the content for each objective. It must be more than a restatement of the objective.	State the time frame for each objective.	List the faculty for each objective.	Describe the teaching methods, strategies, materials, and resources for each objective teaching method/ strategy, materials, resources used for each objective

(Continued)

Continued

Objectives	Content (Topics)	Time Frame	Presenter	Methods
At the completion of this workshop, the learner will:	Pretest	5 minutes	Dr. P. Sagar	Pretest PowerPoint presentation Question and answer
1. Discuss the importance of transcultural nursing.	I. Transcultural nursing Definition Importance of transcultural nursing a. Increase in migration b. Rise in multicultural identities c. Technology vs. cultural values d. Cultural conflicts and clashes e. Increased demand for culturally based health care Brief history of transcultural nursing Cultural assessment guide	20 minutes		Discussion Case studies/ scenarios
2. Analyze the culturally and linguistically appropriate services (CLAS) standards in guiding equitable care.	II. Guidelines Nursing practice CLAS standards Development Themes: Standards 1–3 Standards 47 Interpretation Translation Standards 8–14 Nursing education	10 minutes		

(Continued)

Objectives	Content (Topics)	Time Frame	Presenter	Methods
3. Apply Campinha-Bacote's Biblically Based Model of Cultural Competence in the care of multicultural clients.	III. Campinha-Bacote's Biblically-Based Model of Cultural Competence BASKED Model a. Biblical worldview b. Awareness c. Skill d. Knowledge e. Encounters f. Desire Application of model to care of African Americans Filipino Americans Mexican Americans	25 minutes	Dr. P. Sagar	Case studies/ scenarios Role playing PowerPoint presentation

4. Enumerate culturally competent approaches to patient care.	IV. Cultural competence in client care: Apply Campinha-Bacote's model
	a. Cultural awareness
	b. Cultural knowledge
	  Health-related beliefs
	  Prevalence and incidence of disease
	  Interaction styles
	c. Cultural skill
	  Cultural assessment tools
	d. Cultural encounters
	  Listening
	  Negotiating
	e. Cultural desire
		30 minutes	Dr. P. Sagar	Lecture
				Discussion
				Case studies/ scenarios
				Role playing
				PowerPoint presentation

(Continued)

Continued

Objectives	Content (Topics)	Time Frame	Presenter	Methods
5. Develop strategies to promote cross-cultural communication.	VI. Cultural diversity in the workplace Potential areas of conflict. a. Communication patterns b. Time orientation c. Family obligations d. Space/distance e. Meaning of work Strategies to prevent conflict: a. Mission statement about diversity b. Zero tolerance for discrimination c. Effective cross-cultural communication d. Commitment to multiculturalism at all levels of management	20 minutes		Case studies/ scenarios Role playing PowerPoint presentation Question and answer Posttest Evaluation
	Skill with conflict resolution Some strategies to promote cross cultural communication: a. Pronounce names correctly b. Use proper titles of respect c. Be aware of gender sensitivities	10 minutes		

(Continued)

Objectives	Content (Topics)	Time Frame	Presenter	Methods
	d. Refrain from using derogatory terms e. Avoid words and phrases that may be offensive to others V. Where do we go from here? Follow-up activities Evaluation and post-test			

Proposed 2-hour lesson plan for CE using Campinha-Bacote's Biblically Based Model of Cultural Competence.

Source: Developed from Campinha-Bacote (2005a). *A biblically based model of cultural competence in the delivery of health care services.* Cincinnati, OH: Transcultural C.A.R.E. Associates.

Appendix C

NEW YORK STATE NURSES ASSOCIATION

Educational Activity Overview

Lesson Plan. Using Components Across Models.
STRIVING TOWARD CULTURAL COMPETENCE: A JOURNEY

Purpose: The program is offered to promote cultural competence among health care workers. Attendees will use information in the care of their multicultural clients.

Objectives	Content (Topics)	Time Frame	Presenter	Teaching Methods
Learner oriented with one measurable behavioral verb per objective.	Outline of the content to be covered that will enable the learners to meet their objectives.	State the time frame for each objective.	List the faculty or content expert for each objective.	Describe the teaching methods, strategies, materials, and resources for each objective.

(Continued)

Continued

Objectives	Content (Topics)	Time Frame	Presenter	Teaching Methods

At the completion of this workshop, the learner will:
 	
1. Discuss the importance of cultural competence.
	Pretest
	
	I. Cultural diversity among us
	Some basic concepts
	Culture
	   Cultural shock
	Racism
	Prejudice
	Stereotyping
	Ethnocentrism
	
	Cultural competence:
	  A process
	    Self-reflection and awareness
	    Cultural knowledge
	    Cultural skill
	    Cultural encounters
	    Cultural desire
		5 minutes
		
		15 minutes
			Dr. P. Sagar	Pretest
				PowerPoint presentation
				Question and answer
				AVs
				
				Discussion
				Case studies/ scenarios

2. Critique own cultural assessment guide.	Importance of cultural competence a. Increase in migration b. Rise in multicultural identities c. Technology vs. cultural values d. Increased demand for culturally based health care Cultural assessment guide A close look at your tool. Do you use a theory or framework? Is revision appropriate?	20 minutes	Dr. P. Sagar	Case studies/ scenarios Role playing PowerPoint presentation

(Continued)

Objectives	Content (Topics)	Time Frame	Presenter	Teaching Methods

3. Analyze the culturally and linguistically appropriate services (CLAS) standards in guiding equitable care.	II. Guidelines
	Nursing practice
	  CLAS standards
	   Development
	   Standards 1–3
	   Standards 4¬–7
	    Interpretation
	    Translation
	   Standards 8–14
	Nursing education			

4. Enumerate culturally competent approaches to patient care.	III. Cultural competence in client care
	  A. Cross cultural communication
	  B. Biological variations
	  C. Pain
	  D. Environmental control
	  E. Time and space
	
	IV. Creating a culturally competent organization
	
	Quo Vadis: Where do we go from here?
	Follow-up activities
	  Ongoing approaches to cultural competence
	
	Evaluation and post-test
		15 minutes
		
		5 minutes
			Dr. P. Sagar	PowerPoint presentation
				Discussion
				Case studies/ scenarios:
				  African Americans
				  Mexican Americans
				Role playing
				Clinical examples
				Question and answer
				AVs
				
				Question and answer
				Posttest
				Evaluation

.... And the River Flows

(Dedicated to Madeleine Leininger, founder of Transcultural Nursing)

1

You dug the well of spring with your bare hands
You got trickle of fresh water
The spring barely trickled forth
Yet you persevered. Shadows followed and joined you
all digging deeper.

2

The diggers persisted. You and them
Little streams flowed forth,
seeking the initial flow of the spring
More streams flowed.
Stronger, gathering momentum.

3

Then the river flowed.
I was not there when you dug
I was not there with the helpers
I am now here, gazing at the river.

4

The river flows deep sustaining the fields
And life.
I would help in bringing the water
To all the villages of the world.

Priscilla Limbo Sagar, EdD, ACNS-BC, CTN-A

INDEX